Swing Set Workouts

Karen M. Goeller
Brian Dowd

Swing Set Workouts

ISBN: 978-0-6151-5170-0

Always keep safety in mind!

We were using gravity, gymnastics drills, common exercise movements, and the swing for balance and resistance. As the swing moved further from the normal hanging position it became more resistant and difficult to move, but it provided great resistance for basic and advanced exercise movements. The resistance and movements were smooth and natural, but they were still a great challenge!

Be prepared to compete with gravity during these extreme movements and exercises! You will not believe what can be done with a swing!

Many of the exercises in this book were taken from Karen Goeller's gymnastics training programs. They were drills and conditioning exercises she assigned to her gymnasts in order to help them gain the necessary strength to lift and propel their own body weight. With many of these exercises you will not only gain strength in the specified muscle group, but additional muscle groups will become involved in order to complete the movement. Not only will you gain strength in particular movements, but you will become accustomed to supporting your own body weight. You will become strong in each position required to complete the movements from one supporting position to another.

Other exercises are the more standard exercises that have been seen in the fitness world for many years, but with the use of a swing set.

You will be amazed at the number of exercises Karen has transferred to a swing set all because she went to the beach one day several months ago, saw a swing set, and pictured one exercise, then another, and she continued to imagine several exercises. She took the idea to her nephew, a former college ball player. She challenged him with the exercises, photographed the exercises and completed this project.

Swing Set Workouts

From the gymnastics facility, health club, and boot camp exercises to Karen's swing set fitness. Most people reviewing this book will find several exercises they have never imagined. When you see these exercises and the transition to the swing set you will be tempted to try each and every one of them as soon as you reach the playground. We would not suggest performing all of these exercises in one day, they are much more challenging than you might realize!

Please keep in mind these exercises are not for beginners. By performing these exercises you accept the responsibility for your own personal safety and release the authors, models, and producers of this book from any liability for injuries resulting from the use of this book.

We hope you enjoy this book and wish you the best of luck in reaching your fitness goals!

Always keep safety in mind!

Safety Tips

Make sure the swing set and swing are very secure and stable. They must be in very good condition.

Make sure you do not place your hands on glass, animal droppings, or anything that could cause you harm or illness. Sweep the area prior to use for glass or other dangerous fragments.

Bring a piece of foam or rubber matting for your hands and forearms.

Make sure you will not swing or bump into anyone.

Always hold the chains securely. You could lose your balance and holding the chains may help prevent a fall to the ground.

Only perform these exercises if you have discussed it with your doctor and you are healthy enough to perform strenuous and challenging exercises.

These exercises are challenging. Only perform these exercises if you are able to focus on your safety and technique. Any distractions could be dangerous.

If using a public playground, make sure it is one that allows adults without children. Make sure you follow the rules of the playground and laws in your area.

Wash hands after workout.

Wear sunscreen.

Always keep safety in mind while training!

Contents

Disclaimer

The exercises and advice contained in this book may be too difficult or dangerous for some people. Regardless of your current health status, you should consult with a qualified medical professional to ensure that the exercises and/or workouts in this book are appropriate for your fitness level. The information contained in this book is intended for individuals in good health. Proceed with great caution and at your own risk.

Any activity involving motion or height creates the possibility of accidental injury, paralysis, or death. The instructional materials are intended for use ONLY by properly trained and qualified participants under supervised conditions. Use without proper supervision or coaching could be DANGEROUS and should NOT be undertaken or permitted. Before using, KNOW YOUR LIMITATIONS and the limitations of the equipment you plan to use, including playground equipment. If in doubt always consult a qualified instructor. Always inspect equipment for loose fittings or damage and test for stability before each use.

The writers, models, and producers of this book will not be liable for injuries or consequences sustained in the use of the instructional materials, equipment used, or location.

Swing Set Workouts

Always keep safety in mind!

General Fitness Workout 1

There is one exercise per body area in this workout. This workout has been created to help the user gain and maintain a good general fitness level for daily activity. There are six exercises in this workout, but don't be fooled, it is not an easy workout!

Three sets per exercise are recommended and 10-15 repetitions per set are appropriate for this type of workout.

Swing Set Workouts

Always keep safety in mind!

Squat – Hold Swing (Lean Back)

Start facing the swing. Grasp the outer portion of the swing with both hands and wrap fingers over the swing. (Other option is to grasp the lowest portion of the chains.) Holding the swing securely, lean backward and walk your feet forward so that you are at approximately a 45 degree angle. Make sure your feet will not slide. Keep your chest up and bend both knees to perform a squat. Make sure your knees remain in line with your hips. Do not allow your knees to fall toward each other. Make sure your knees do not go forward beyond your toes. Straighten and bend your knees for the desired number of repetitions.

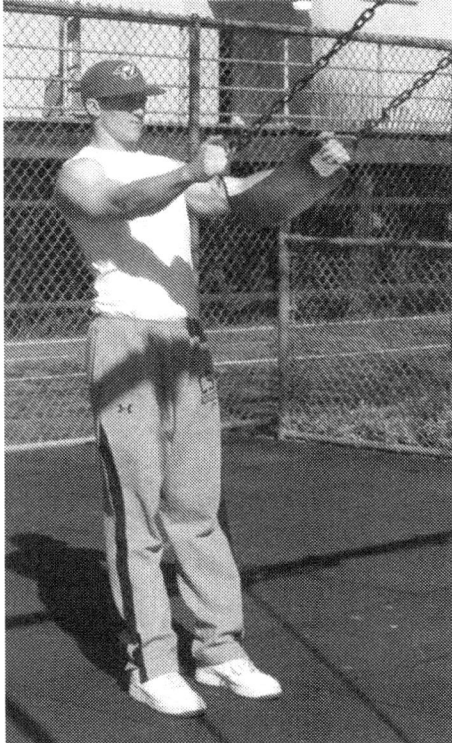

Swing Set Workouts

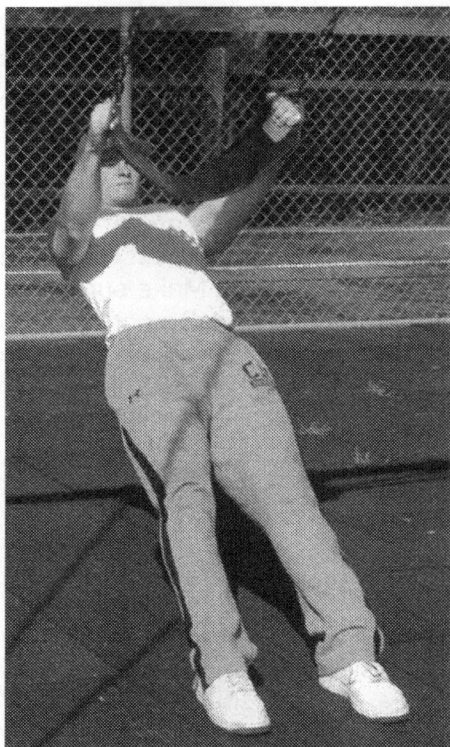

Always keep safety in mind!

General Fitness Workout 1

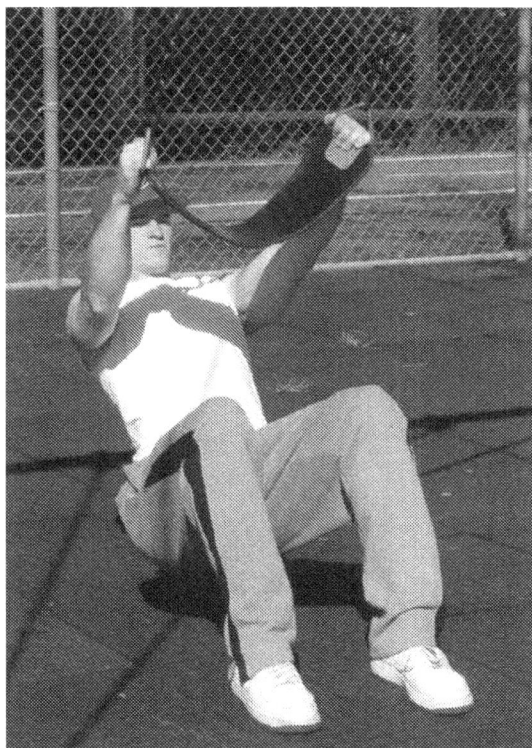

Swing Set Workouts

Modified Pull Up – High

Grasp the outer portion of the swing with both hands and wrap fingers over the swing. Keeping your fingers wrapped around the bottom of the swing, lean backward and move your feet forward so that you are at a slight angle. Make sure your feet will not slide. Next, pull your chest in towards the swing. Keep your body straight throughout this exercise. You should feel this in your back and biceps.

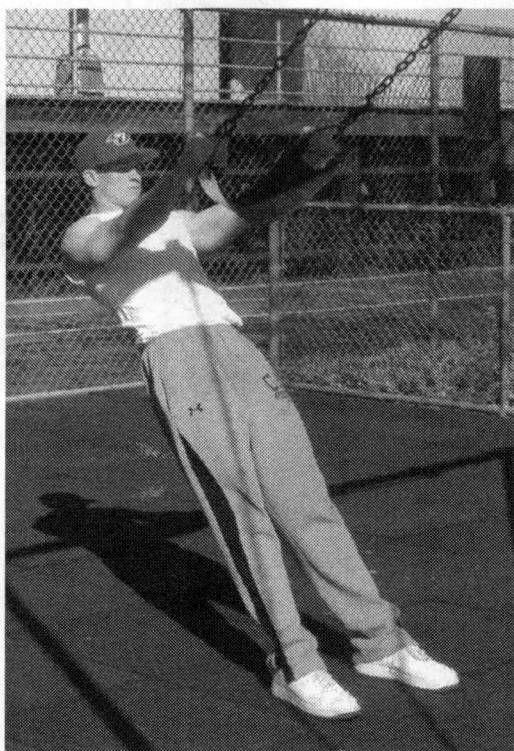

Always keep safety in mind!

General Fitness Workout 1

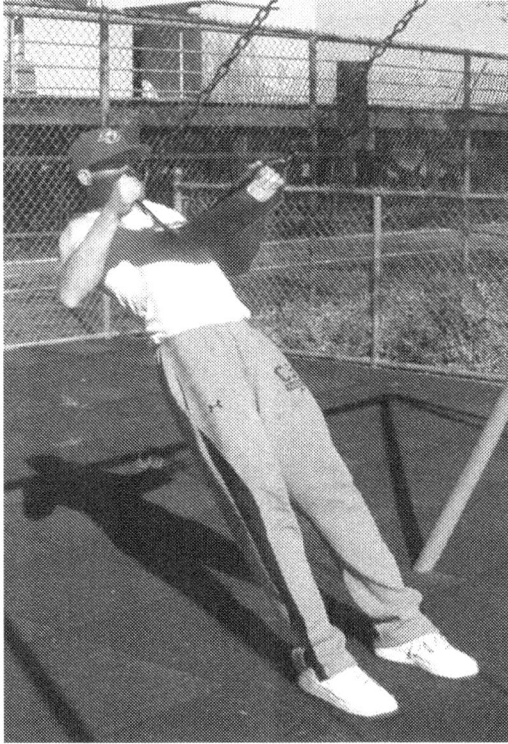

Swing Set Workouts

Swing Walks - Forward and Back

Start with your back facing the swing. Place your hands on the ground. Next, place your shins on the swing. You should be in a push up / plank position with your shins on the swing. Keep your arms straight throughout the exercise. Walk your hands forward as far as possible and then walk backward as far as possible. You will be pulling forward using your back / latissimus muscles and pushing backward using your shoulders. It will be slightly more difficult than the swing rocks because you will be pulling and pushing with one the muscles on one side at a time. You will also be supporting your body with one side at a time as you shift your weight from one hand to the other. You should feel this in your chest, shoulders, back, triceps, and core muscles. Repeat the swing walks for the desired number of repetitions.

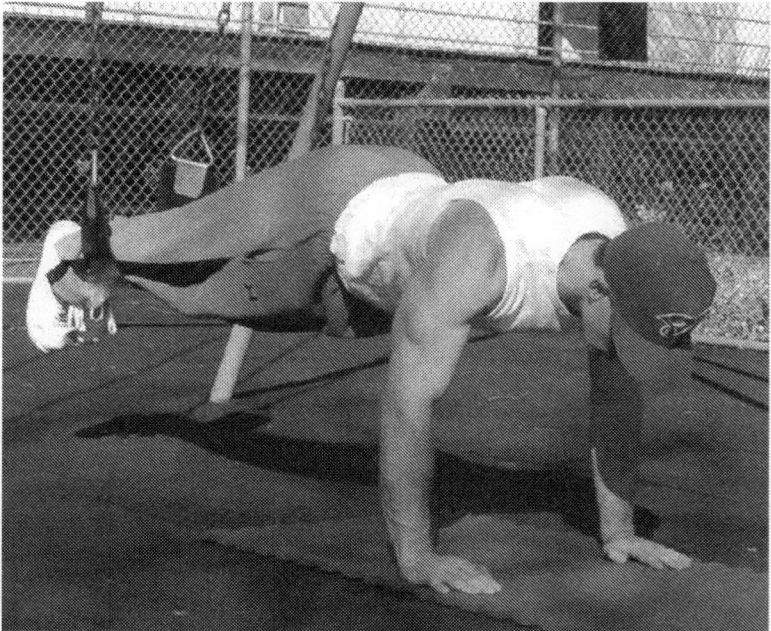

Always keep safety in mind!

General Fitness Workout 1

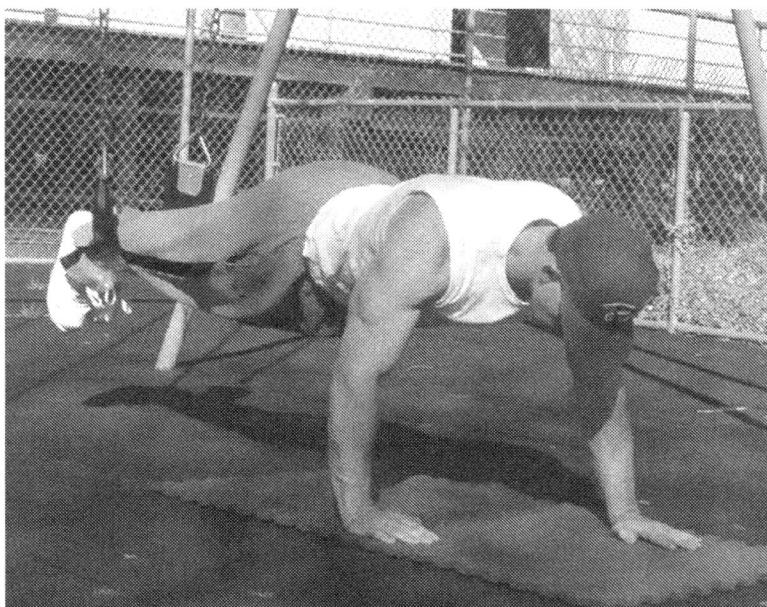

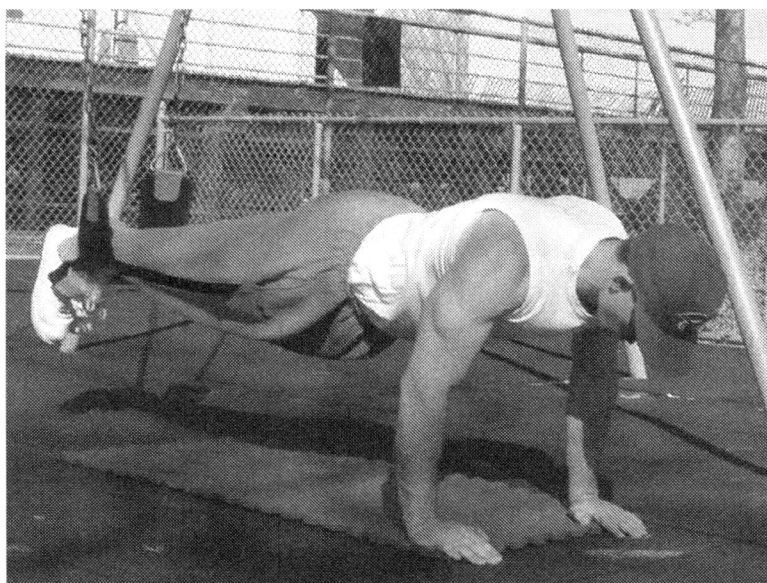

Swing Set Workouts

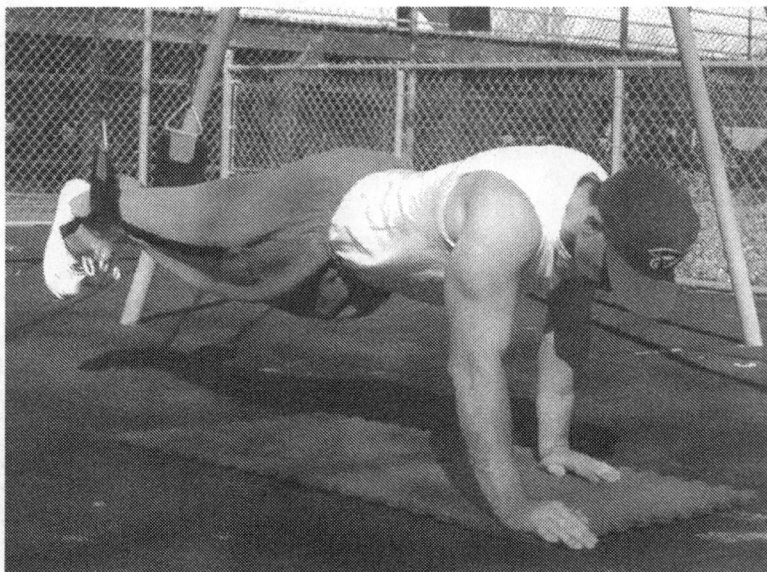

Always keep safety in mind!

General Fitness Workout 1

Alternate this exercise with Flutter Kicks. Perform 10 Double Crunches, 10 Flutter Kicks, and 10 Double Crunches. This will give you 30 abdominal repetitions. Perform of the repetitions nonstop if you are able.

Double Crunch

Sit on the swing, hold the chains, and lean back. Lift both legs in front of your body to hip /swing height. Once both legs are at hip / swing height, bring both knees in toward your chest together. As you bring your knees in toward your chest, sit up to allow your chest and knees to meet. Once your knees and chest have formed a tuck position, return to the starting position. Continue to bring your knees in and chest up for the desired number of repetitions. You should feel this in your abdominal and hip flexor muscles.

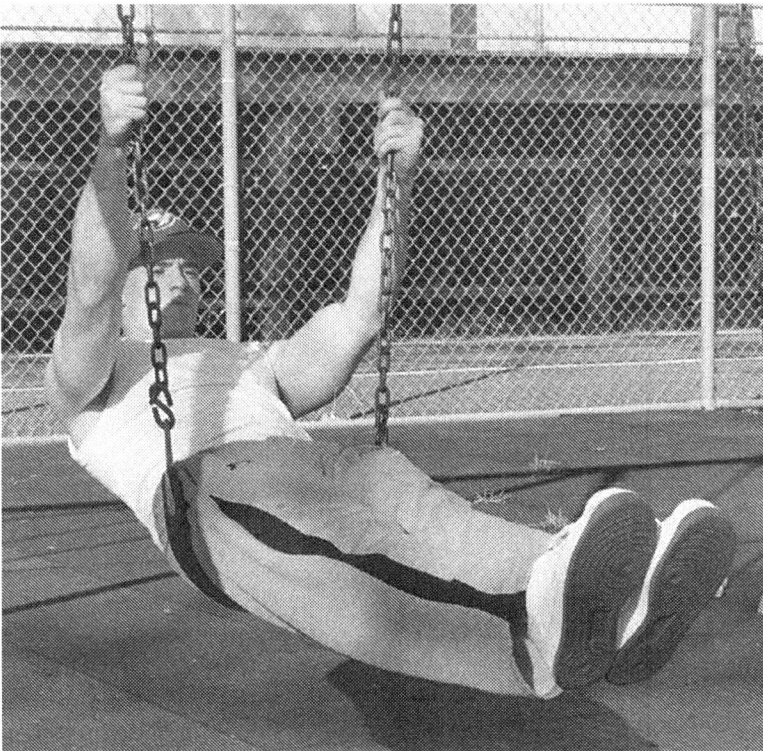

Swing Set Workouts

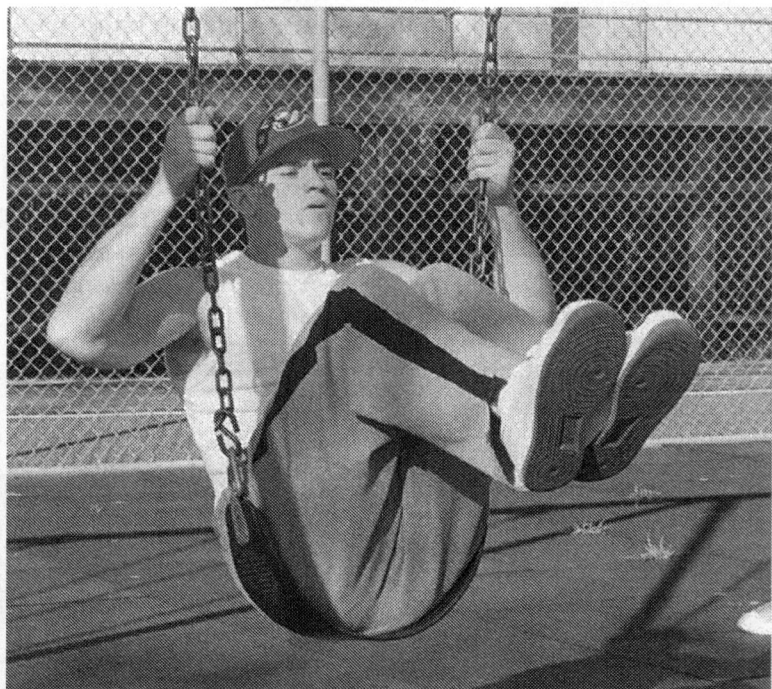

Always keep safety in mind!

General Fitness Workout 1

Flutter Kicks

Sit on the swing, hold the chains, and lean back.
Keeping your legs straight, lift them in front of your
body to hip / swing height. Once both legs are at hip /
swing height, lift your right leg up 6-8 inches. Next,
simultaneously return the right leg to hip / swing height
and lift the left leg 6-8 inches off the swing. Continue
to perform very quick alternating low lifts for the
desired number of repetitions. Keep your legs straight
throughout the exercise. You should feel this in your
abdominal and hip flexor muscles.

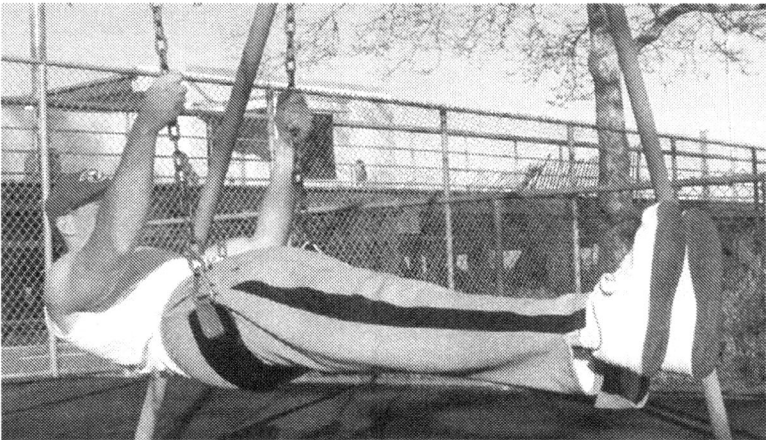

Swing Set Workouts

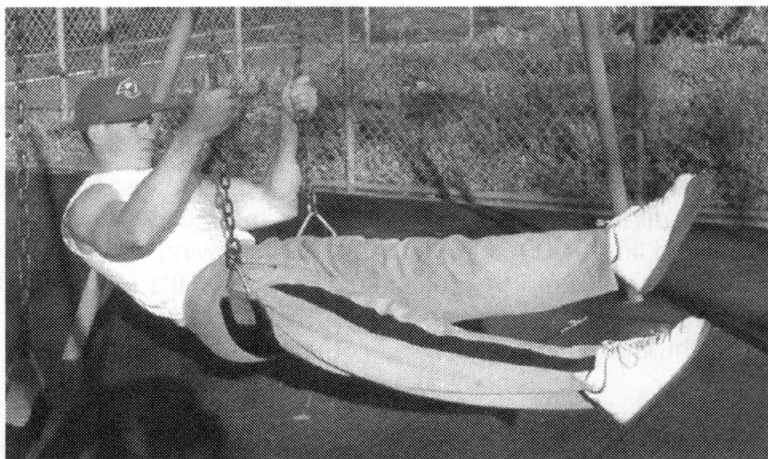

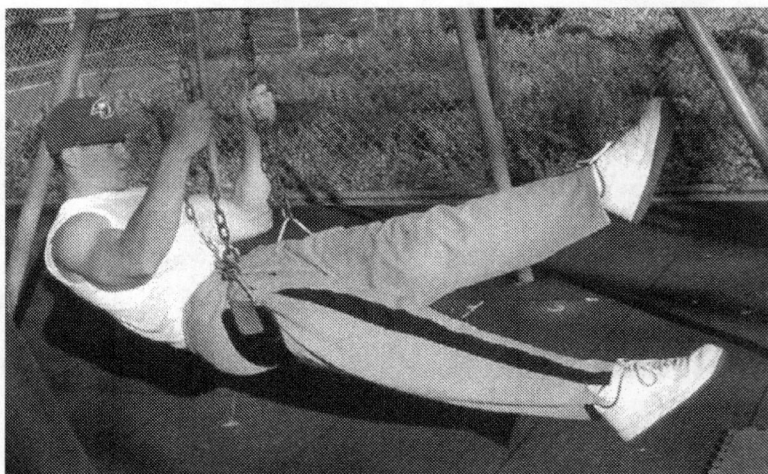

Always keep safety in mind!

General Fitness Workout 2

There is one exercise per body area in this workout. This workout has been created to help the user gain and maintain a good general fitness level for daily activity. This workout is time efficient and has been created to produce results!

Three sets per exercise are recommended and 10-15 repetitions per set are appropriate for this type of workout.

Swing Set Workouts

Always keep safety in mind!

General Fitness Workout 2

Supported Leg Press

Start lying with your upper back on swing and hands on chains. Begin with your legs straight and your body at approximately a 45 degree angle. Your body should be in a straight line form head to toe. Once positioned, bend your knees until they form a 90 degree angle. Your upper body continues to be supported by the swing. Make sure your knees remain in line with your hips. Do not allow your knees to fall toward each other. Make sure your knees do not go forward beyond your toes. Straighten and bend your knees for the desired number of repetitions.

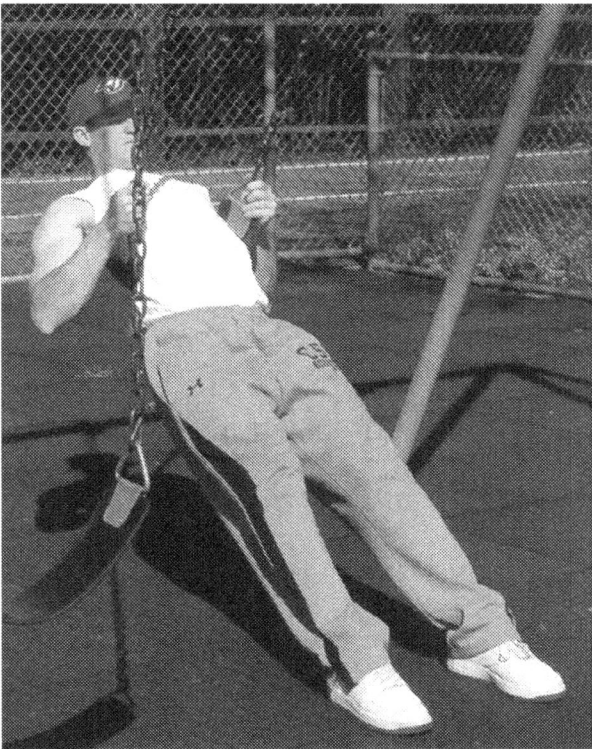

Swing Set Workouts

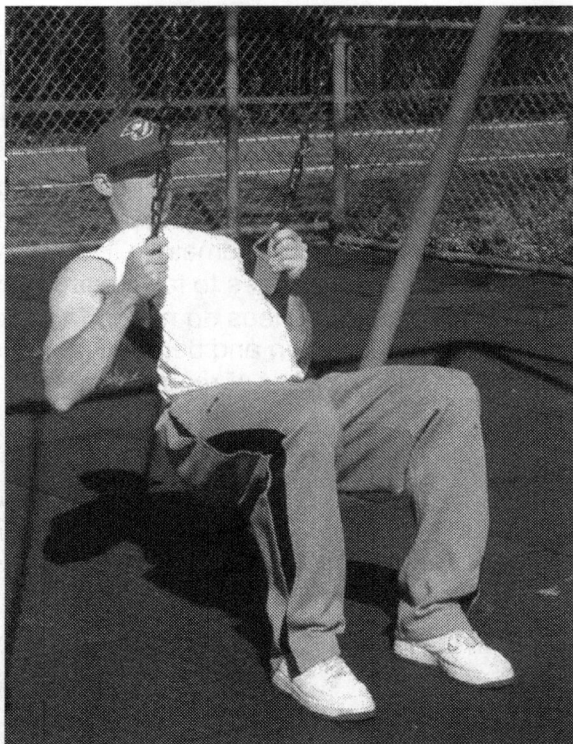

Always keep safety in mind!

Modified Pull Up – Low

Grasp the outer portion of the swing with both hands and wrap fingers over the swing. Keeping your fingers wrapped around the bottom of the swing, lean backwards and walk your feet forward so that you are at a low position. Make sure your feet will not slide. Next, pull your chest in toward the swing. Keep your body straight throughout this exercise. You should feel this in your back and biceps.

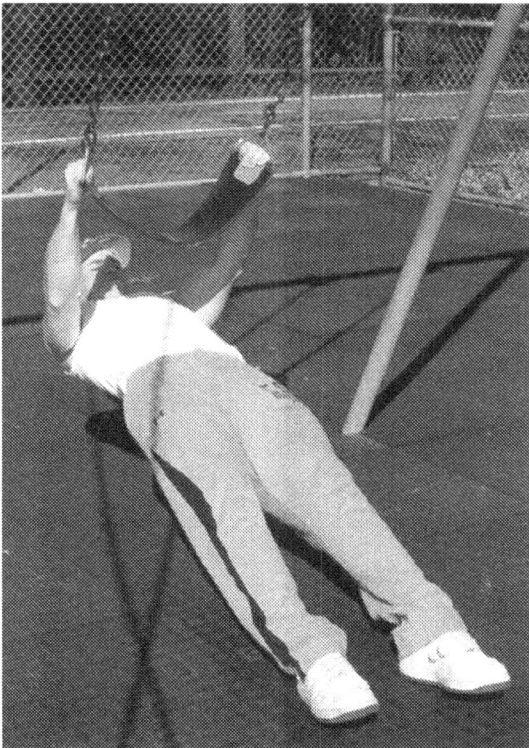

Swing Set Workouts

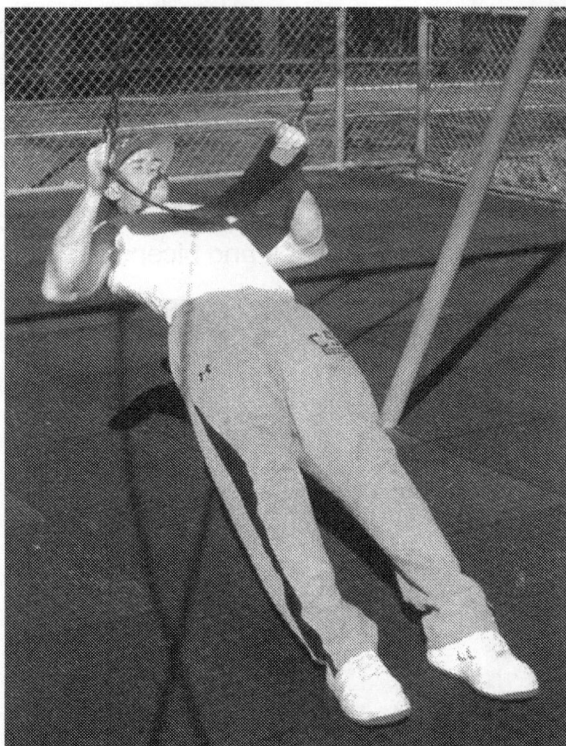

Always keep safety in mind!

Swing Push Ups – Shins on Swing
Start with your back facing the swing. Place your hands on the ground. Next, place your shins on the swing. You should be in a push up position with your shins on the swing. Once positioned, lower your chest and chin near the ground and then push back up. Keep your core muscles tight and do not allow your lower back to hang down. Repeat for the desired number of repetitions. You should feel this in your chest, triceps, and core muscles.

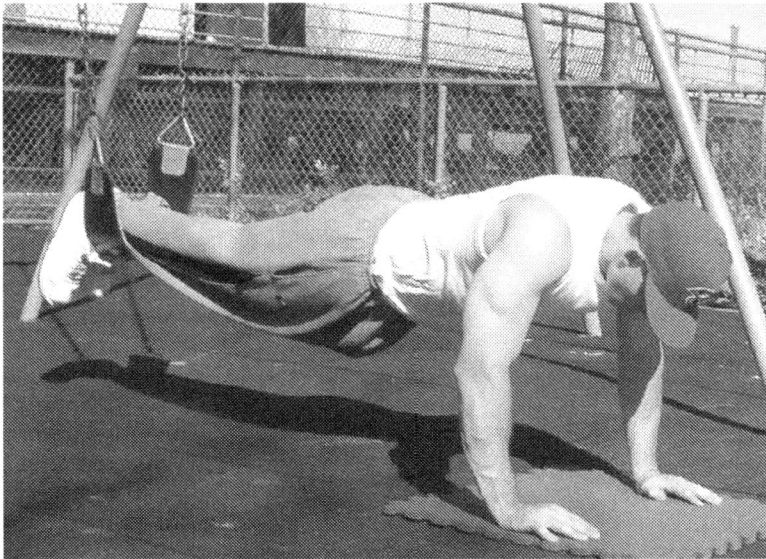

Swing Set Workouts

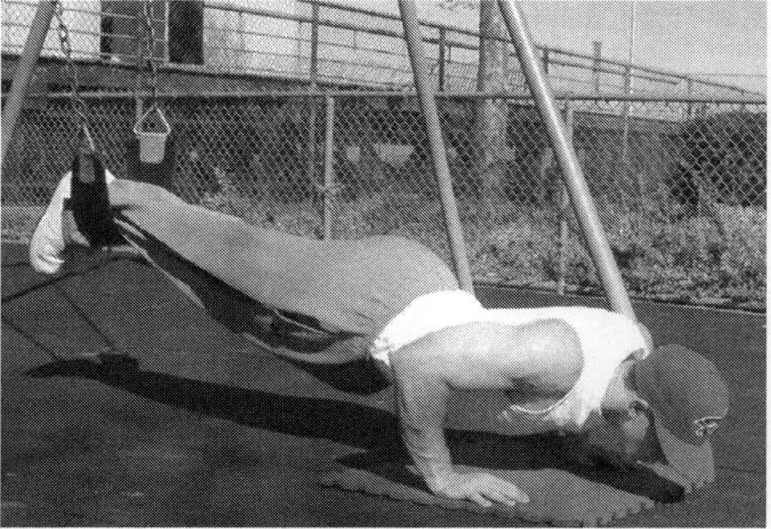

Always keep safety in mind!

Biceps Curl -Narrow

Grasp the bottom of the swing with both hands and wrap your fingers over the swing. The small fingers on each hand should be near each other to form a narrow grip. Keep your fingers wrapped around the bottom of the swing securely. Lean backwards so that your arms start nearly straight and walk your feet forward so that you are standing at a 45 degree angle. Make sure your feet will not slide. Next, using your biceps pull your chest in towards the swing. Keep your body straight and elbows near your ribs throughout this exercise. Keep your shoulders still while pulling so that you are performing a bicep curl, not a pull up. Open your arms and repeat the curl for the desired number of repetitions. You should feel this in your biceps.

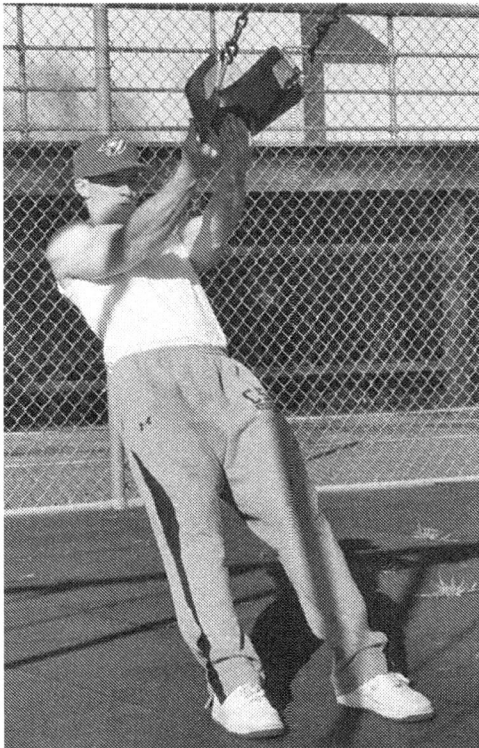

Swing Set Workouts

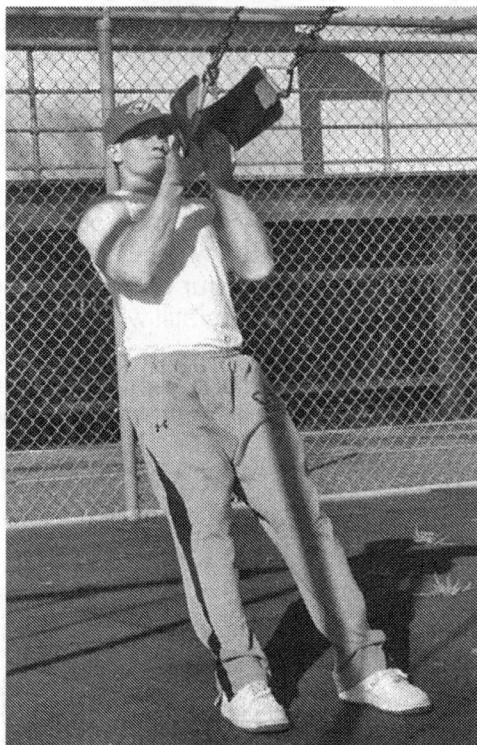

Always keep safety in mind!

General Fitness Workout 2

Alternate this exercise with Knee Ins. Perform 10 Belly Squeezes, 10 Knee Ins, and 10 Belly Squeezes. This will give you 30 abdominal repetitions. Perform of the repetitions nonstop if you are able.

Belly Squeeze

Start with your back facing the swing. Place your hands on the ground. Next, place your shins on the swing. You should be in a push up position with your shins on the swing. Next, pull your abdominal muscles in so that you slightly bend at the hips to form a small pike position. Return to the straight push / plank position and repeat the lift for the desired number of repetitions. Think of lifting the abdominal section near your ribs rather than your hips with this exercise. You should feel this in your core muscles.

This exercise can be performed on your forearms to change the angle and muscle demand. It is also a great alternative if your wrists are sore.

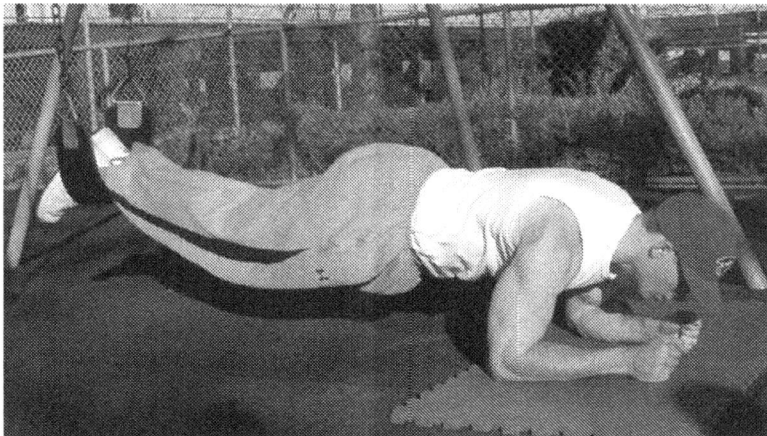

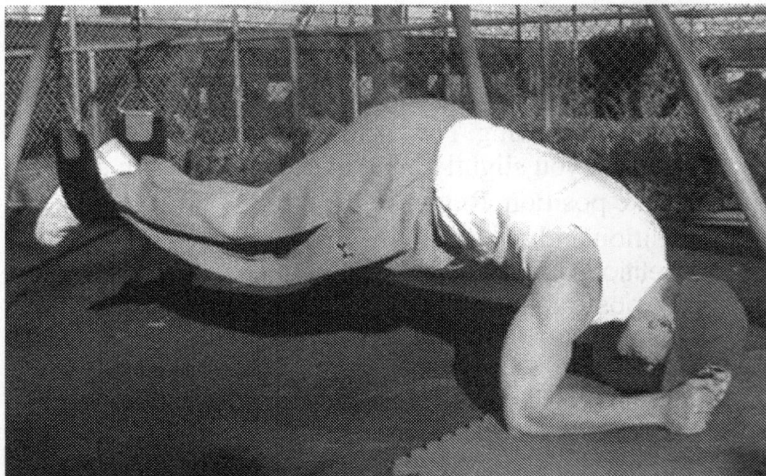

Always keep safety in mind!

Knee In - Tuck

Start with your back facing the swing. Place your hands on the ground. Next, place your shins on the swing. You should be in a push up / plank position with your shins on the swing. Next, pull your knees toward your chest, bending at the hips to form a tuck position. Your hips will be slightly higher than your head and your thighs should be touching your ribs. Your arms will remain straight. Return to the straight push / plank position and repeat the knee tuck for the desired number of repetitions. You should feel this in your core, chest, and shoulder muscles.

This exercise can be performed on your forearms to change the angle and muscle demand. It is also a great alternative if your wrists are sore.

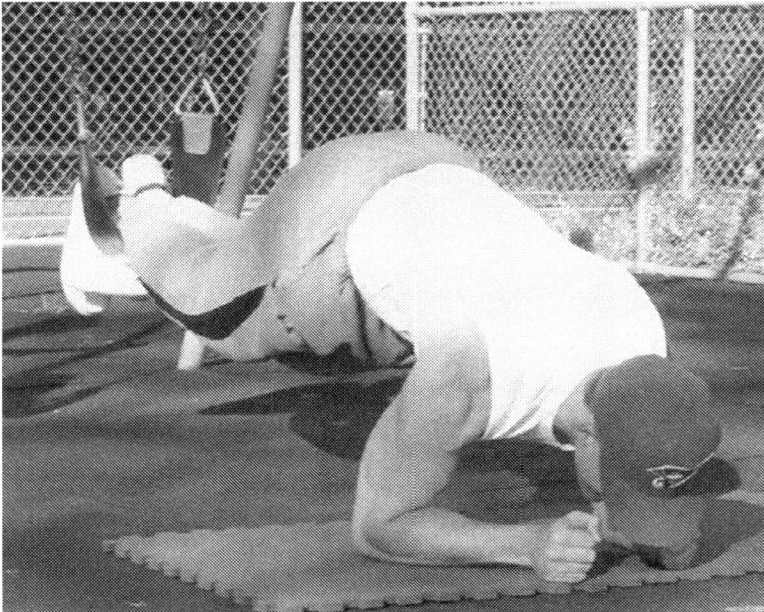

Swing Set Workouts

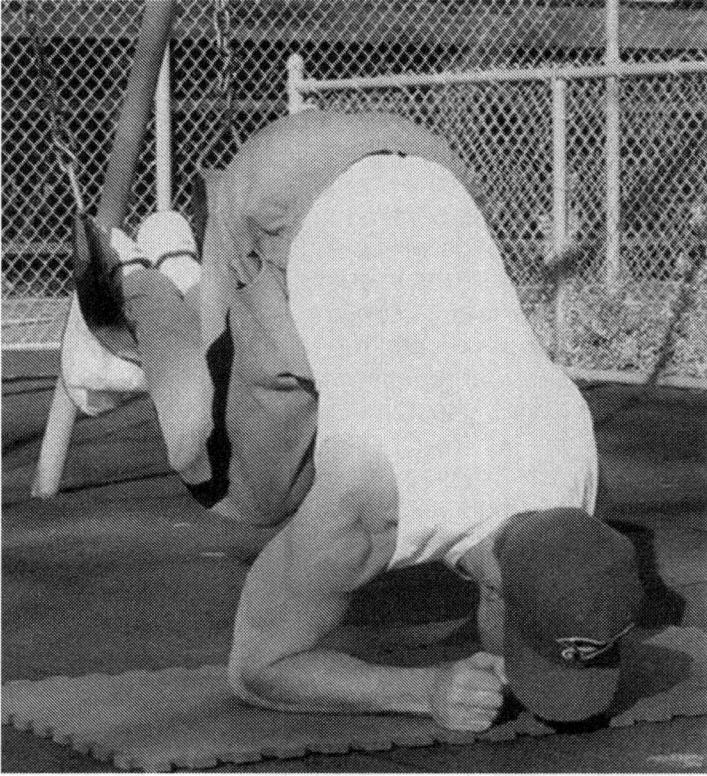

Always keep safety in mind!

General Fitness Workout 3

There is at least one exercise per body area in this workout. This workout has been created to help the user gain and maintain a high general fitness level. There are five exercises in this workout. Don't be fooled, the exercises are not easy and this is not an easy workout!

Three sets per exercise are recommended and 10-15 repetitions per set are appropriate for this type of workout.

Swing Set Workouts

Always keep safety in mind!

Bulgarian Squat

Start with your back facing the swing. Lift your right foot up behind your body to place your right shin on the swing. Allow the swing to slightly move backward. Once you are balanced with your right shin on the swing, bend your left leg to perform a single leg squat. Make sure you keep your left knee in line with the hip and the toes on that side. Make sure you do not allow your knee to move forward, beyond your toes. Keep your chest up throughout the exercise.

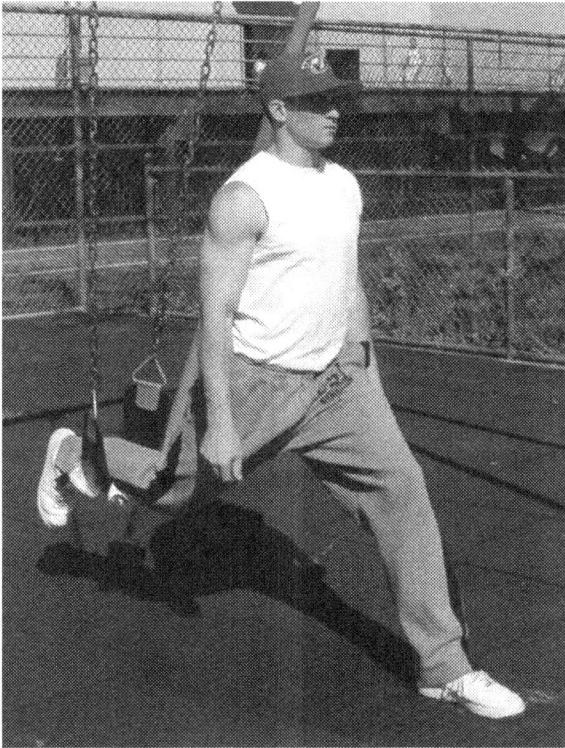

Swing Set Workouts

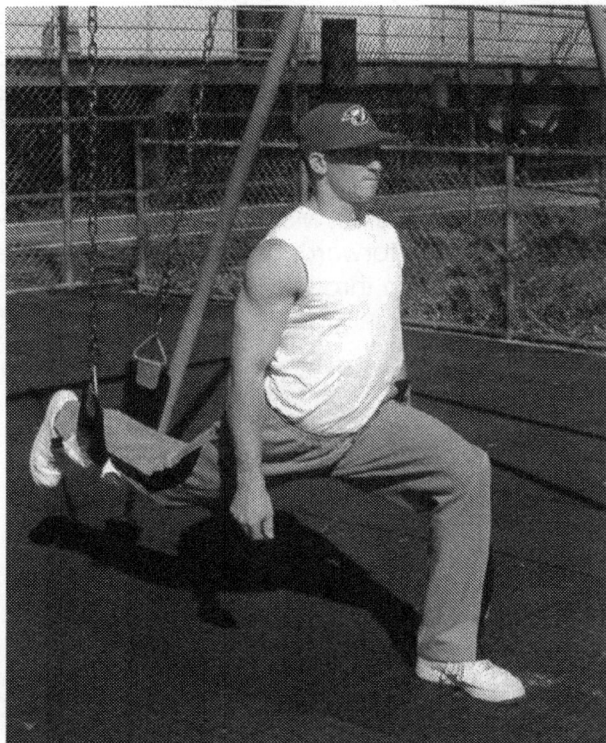

Always keep safety in mind!

Calf Raise

Start facing the swing. Grasp the center of the swing with both hands. Keeping your fingers wrapped around the bottom of the swing, walk your feet backwards so that you are at an angle. Once in position, lift your heels off the ground. Return to the starting position. Continue to lift your heels for the desired number of repetitions. Keep your chest up and your body straight throughout this exercise.

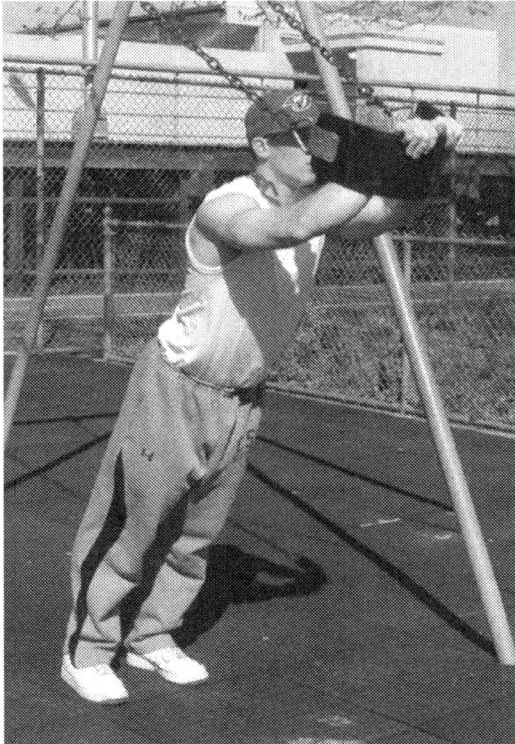

Swing Set Workouts

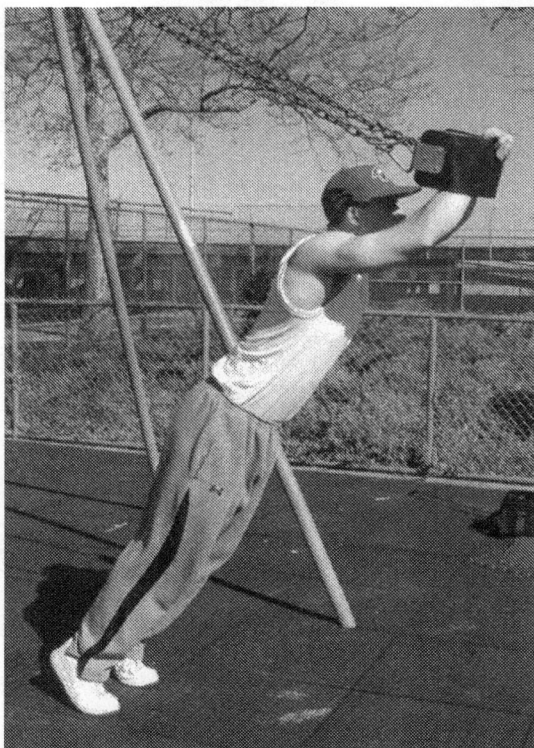

Always keep safety in mind!

Straight Arm Lat Pull Down

Grasp the swing with both hands and position palms near the outer edge of swing. Keeping your fingers wrapped around the swing, raise the swing forward and up so that your arms are up by your ears. Your body will remain straight throughout this exercise. Lean forward and allow the swing to help with balance. Walk your feet backwards so that you are at an angle. Next, lower the swing forward and down so that the swing is below your ribs. Bring the swing back above your head and lower the swing again. You should feel this in your back, chest, and core muscles. It is similar to a straight arm dumbbell pullover or a kip motion.

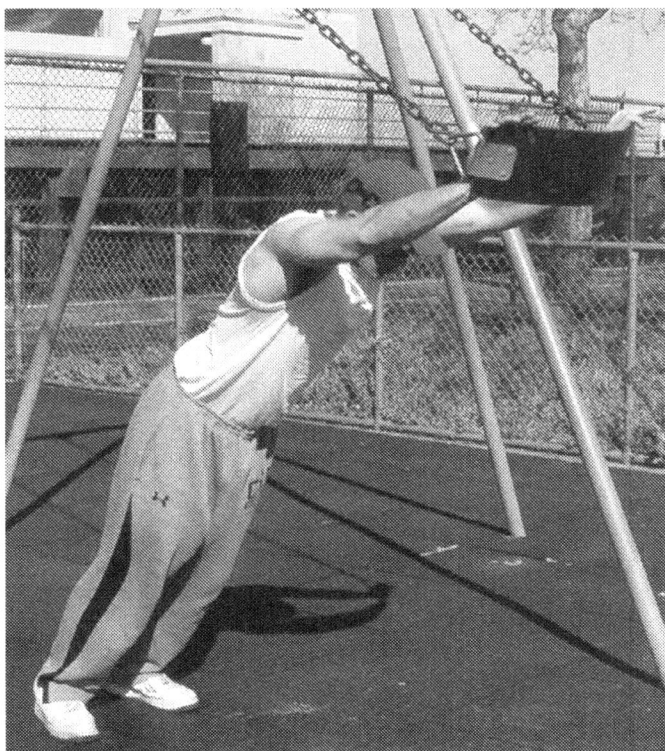

Swing Set Workouts

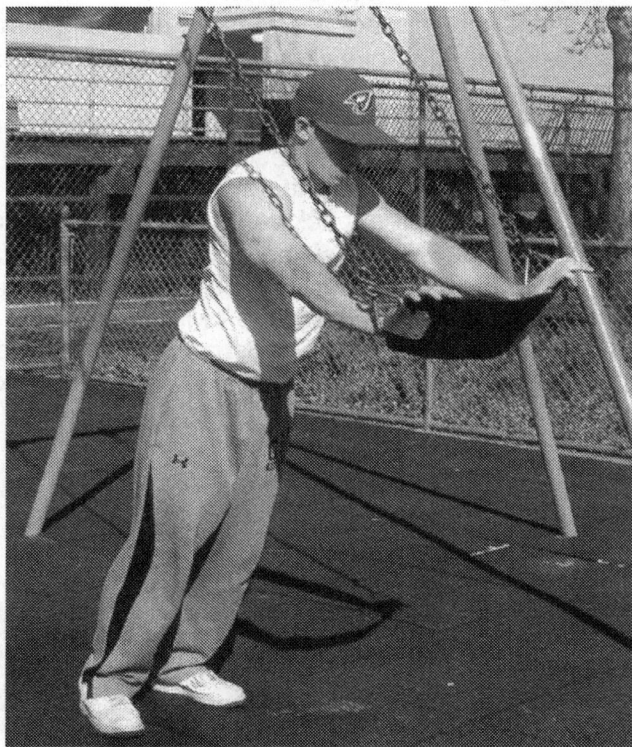

Always keep safety in mind!

General Fitness Workout 3

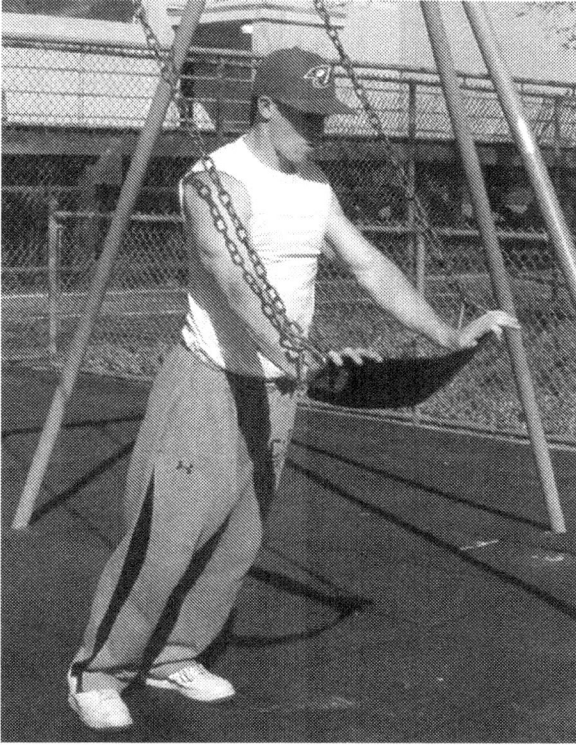

Pike / Virtual Handstand Push Up

Start with your back facing the swing. Place your hands on the ground. Next, place your shins on the swing. You should be in a push up / plank position with your shins on the swing. Next, pull your belly in so that you bend at the hips to form a full pike position, virtual handstand. Your hips will be directly above your head. Once in the virtual handstand, bend your elbows so that your head moves towards the ground. Do not allow your head to touch the ground! Your legs will remain straight. Your upper body will be in a virtual handstand during these push ups. Return to the virtual handstand and then to the straight push up / plank position. Repeat the handstand pushup for the desired number of repetitions. You should feel this in your shoulders and core muscles.

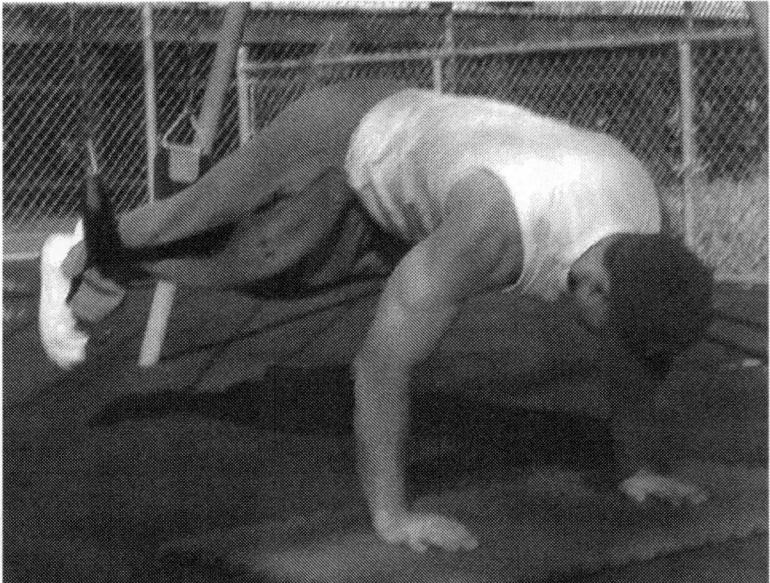

General Fitness Workout 3

Do not allow your head or face to contact the ground.
Only perform this exercise of you are strong enough to
support yourself upside down.

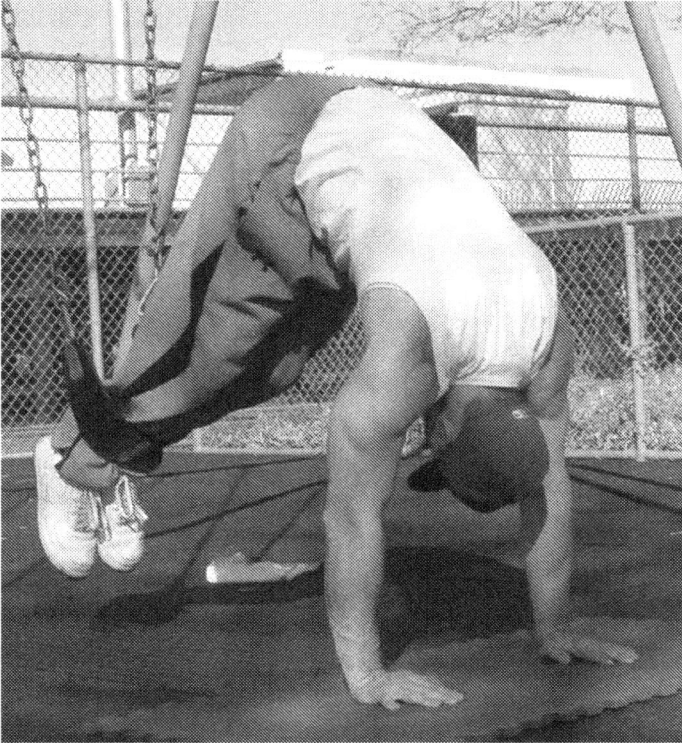

Swing Set Workouts

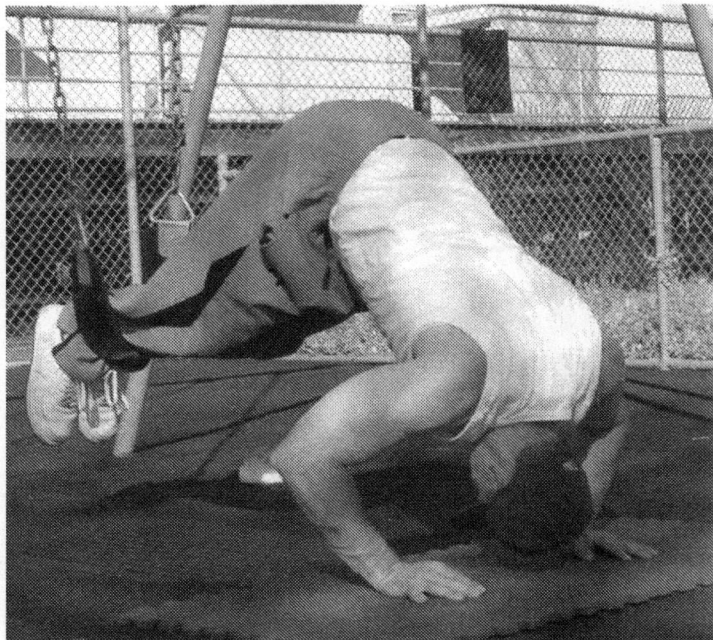

Always keep safety in mind!

Biceps Curl - Narrow

Grasp the bottom of the swing with both hands and wrap your fingers over the swing. The small fingers on each hand should be near each other to form a narrow grip. Keep your fingers wrapped around the bottom of the swing securely. Lean backwards so that your arms start nearly straight and walk your feet forward so that you are standing at a 45 degree angle. Make sure your feet will not slide. Next, using your biceps pull your chest in towards the swing. Keep your body straight and elbows near your ribs throughout this exercise. Keep your shoulders still while pulling so that you are performing a bicep curl, not a pull up. Open your arms and repeat the curl for the desired number of repetitions. You should feel this in your biceps.

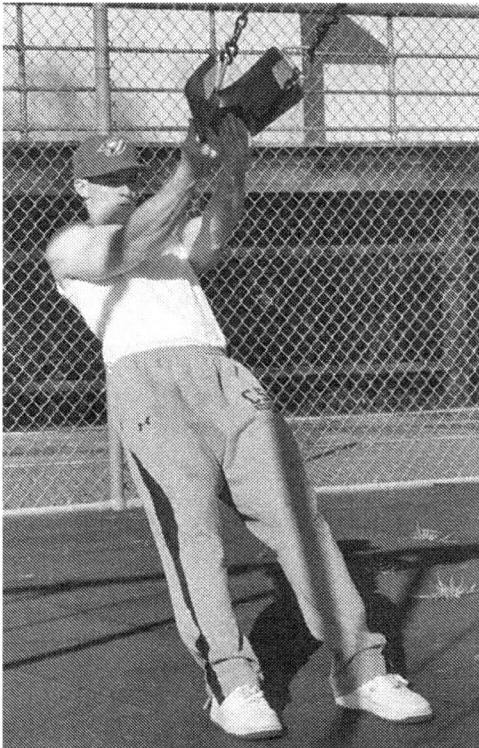

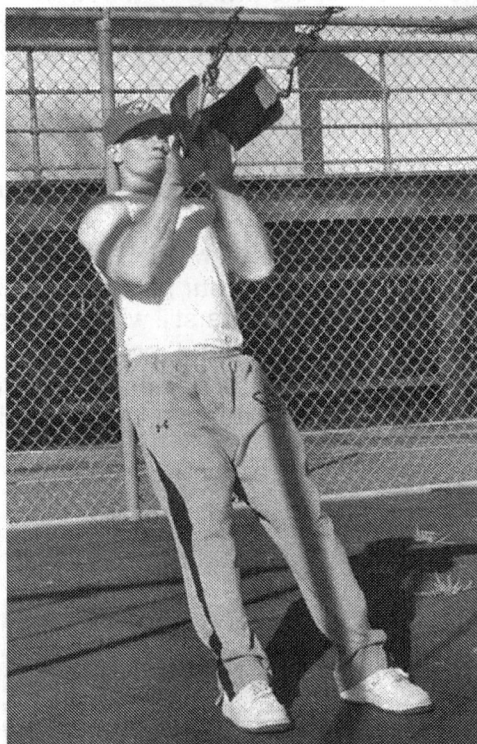

Always keep safety in mind!

General Fitness Workout 3

Push Up Alternate Lifts - Shins on Swing

Start with your back facing the swing. Place your hands on the ground. Next, place your shins / ankles on the swing. You should be in a push up / plank position with your shins on the swing. Lift your right hand and your left leg up simultaneously. Return your right hand to the ground and left leg to the swing then repeat the motion with your left hand and right leg. Your arms and legs remain straight. Keep your back straight and core muscles tight. Repeat the alternate lifts for the desired number of repetitions. You should feel this in your core muscles.

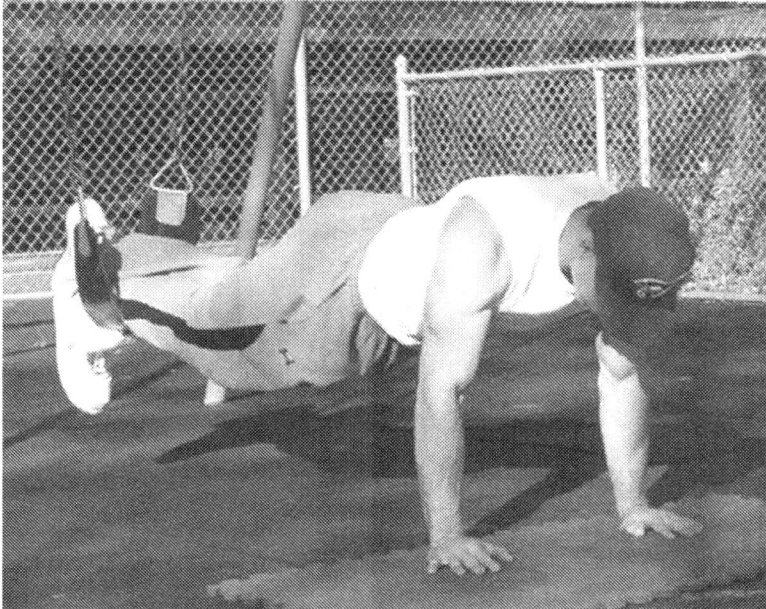

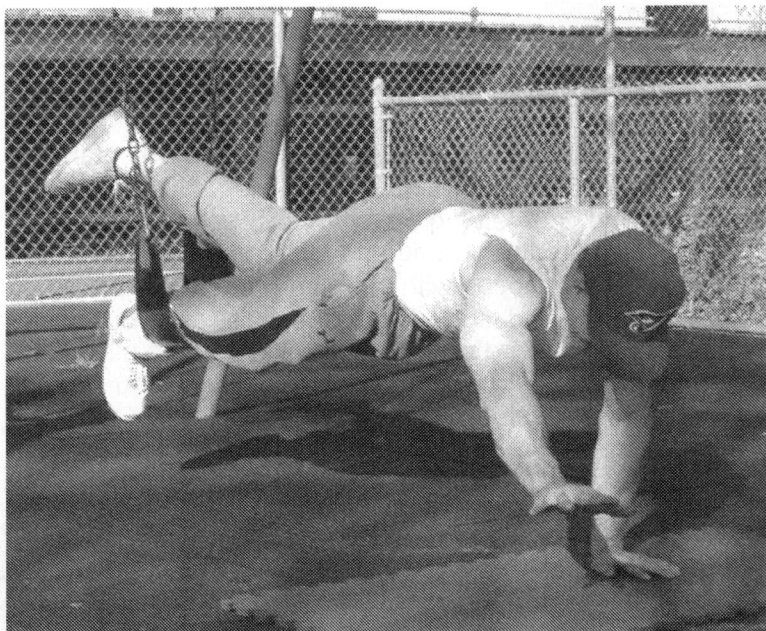

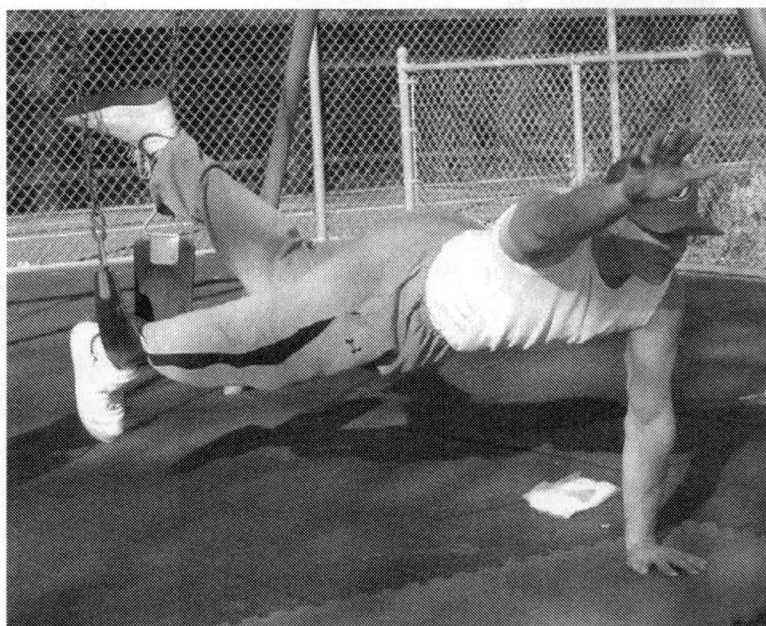

Always keep safety in mind!

Advanced Full Body Workout 1

If you enjoy a good challenge and working up a sweat, this workout is for you! There are nine exercises in this workout.

Two to three sets per exercise are recommended and 10-15 repetitions per set are appropriate for this type of workout.

Swing Set Workouts

Always keep safety in mind!

Advanced Full Body Workout 1

Squat – Hold Swing (Lean Back)

Start facing the swing. Grasp the outer portion of the swing with both hands and wrap fingers over the swing. (Other option is to grasp the lowest portion of the chains.) Holding the swing securely, lean backward and walk your feet forward so that you are at approximately a 45 degree angle. Make sure your feet will not slide. Keep your chest up and bend both knees to perform a squat. Make sure your knees remain in line with your hips. Do not allow your knees to fall toward each other. Make sure your knees do not go forward beyond your toes. Straighten and bend your knees for the desired number of repetitions.

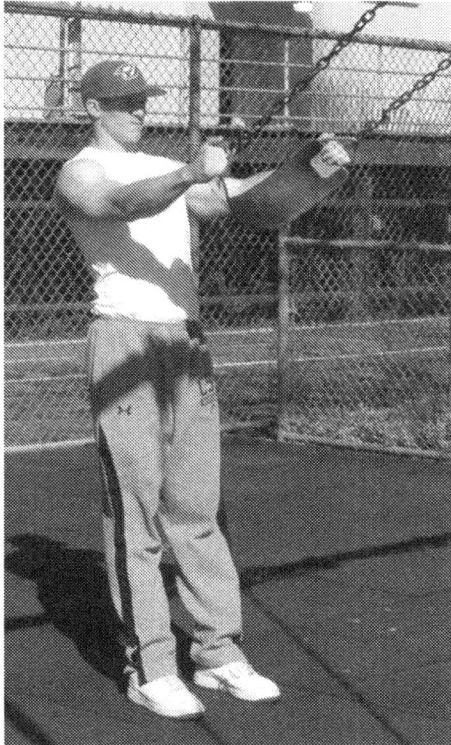

Swing Set Workouts

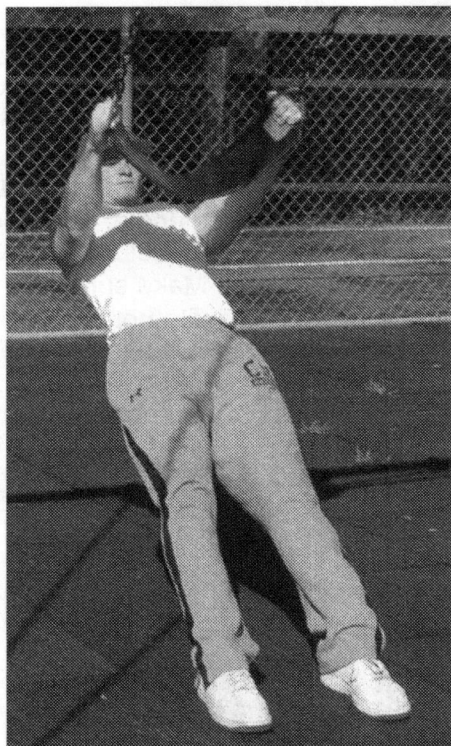

Always keep safety in mind!

Advanced Full Body Workout 1

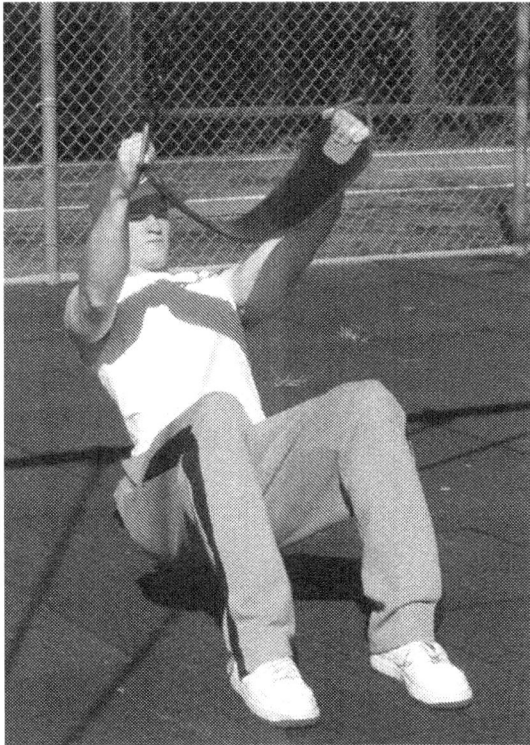

Swing Set Workouts

Single Leg Swing Squat – Hold Swing
Start facing the swing. Grasp the outer portion of the swing with both hands and wrap fingers over the swing. Holding the swing securely, lean backward and walk your feet forward so that you are at approximately a 45 degree angle. Make sure your feet will not slide. Lift your right foot off the ground and hold the straight leg up in front of your body. Keep your chest up and bend your left knee to perform a single leg squat. Make sure you keep your left knee in line with your left hip and toes. Make sure you do not allow your knee to bend to far forward beyond your toes. Straighten and bend your knee for the desired number of repetitions. Perform this exercise for the same number of repetitions with your other leg.

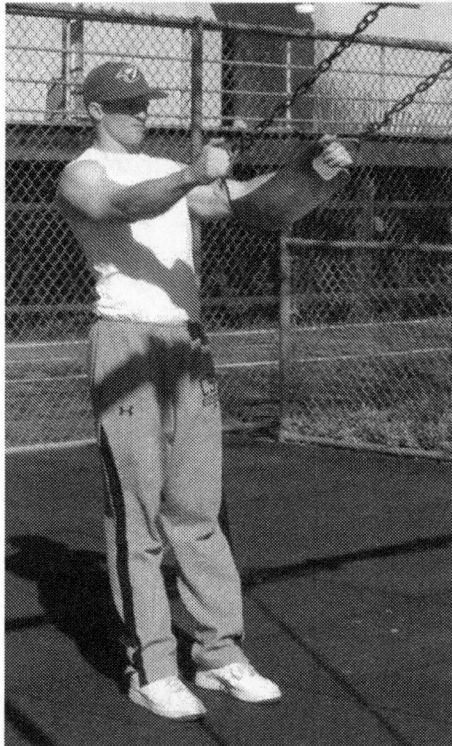

Always keep safety in mind!

Advanced Full Body Workout 1

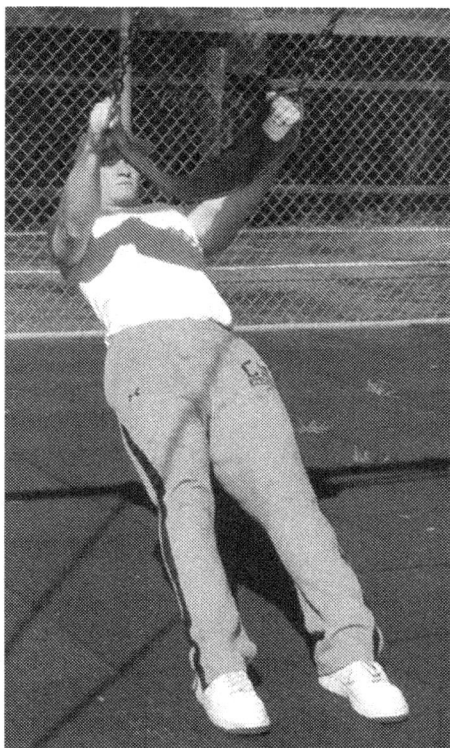

Swing Set Workouts

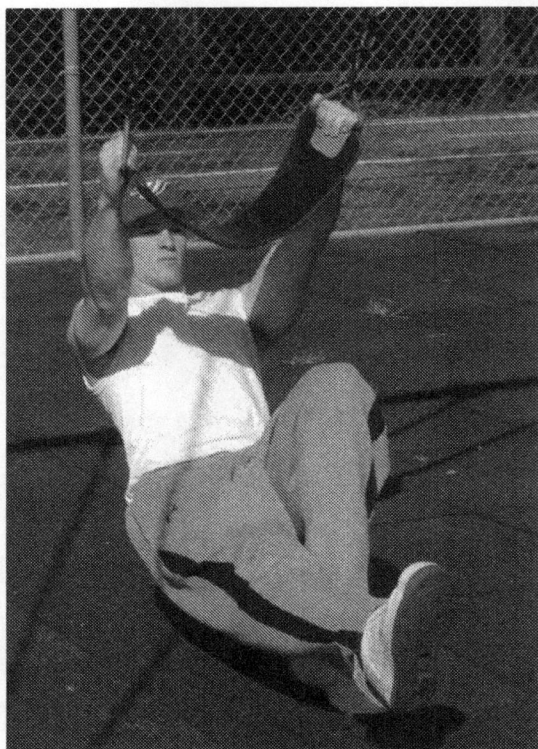

Always keep safety in mind!

Advanced Full Body Workout 1

Modified Pull Up – Low

Grasp the outer portion of the swing with both hands and wrap fingers over the swing. Keeping your fingers wrapped around the bottom of the swing, lean backwards and walk your feet forward so that you are at a low position. Make sure your feet will not slide. Next, pull your chest in toward the swing. Keep your body straight throughout this exercise. You should feel this in your back and biceps.

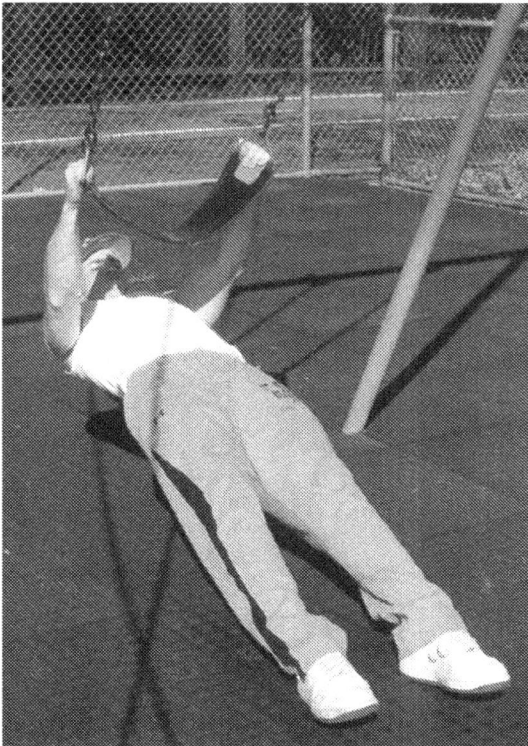

Swing Set Workouts

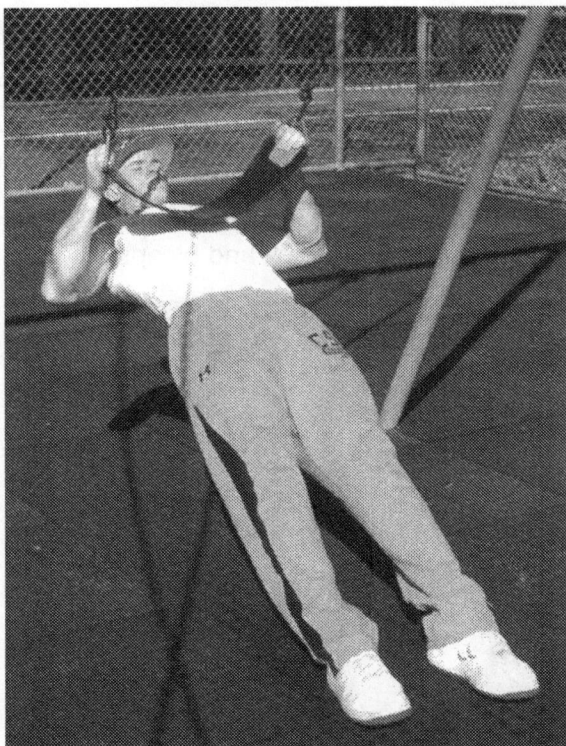

Always keep safety in mind!

Advanced Full Body Workout 1

Straight Arm Lat Pull Down

Grasp the swing with both hands and position palms near the outer edge of swing. Keeping your fingers wrapped around the swing, raise the swing forward and up so that your arms are up by your ears. Your body will remain straight throughout this exercise.

Lean forward and allow the swing to help with balance. Walk your feet backwards so that you are at an angle. Next, lower the swing forward and down so that the swing is below your ribs. Bring the swing back above your head and lower the swing again. You should feel this in your back, chest, and core muscles. It is similar to a straight arm dumbbell pullover or a kip motion.

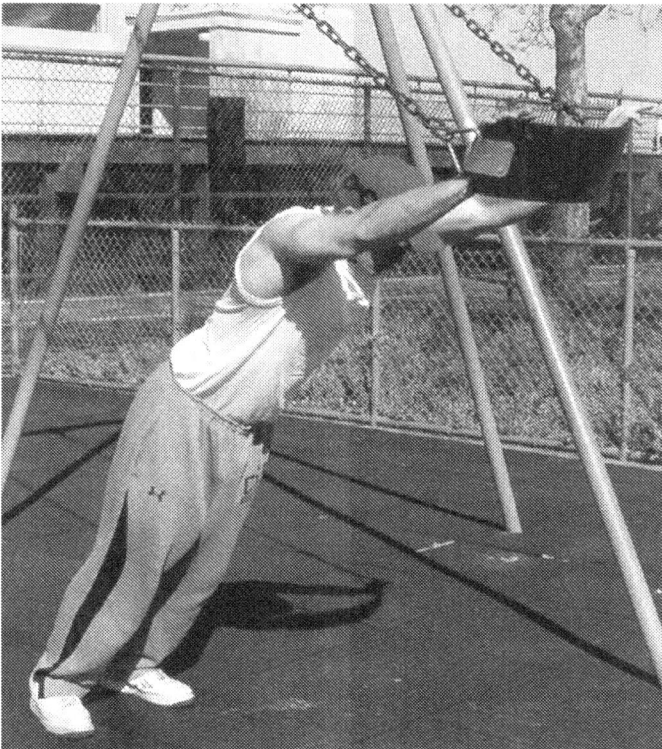

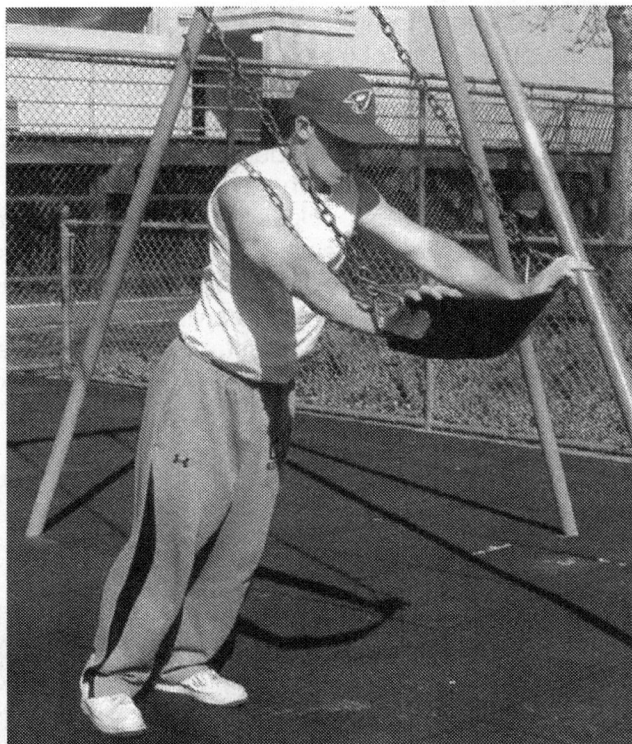

Always keep safety in mind!

Advanced Full Body Workout 1

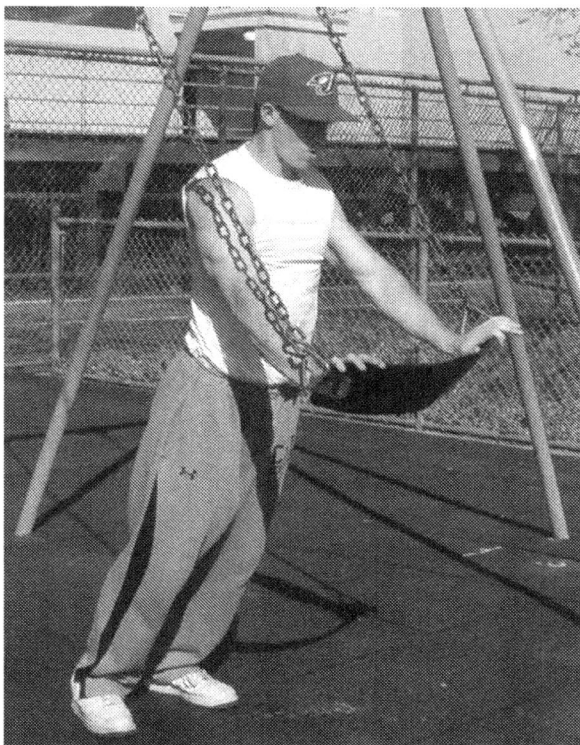

Swing Rocks / Pulls with Push Up

Start with your back facing the swing. Place your hands on the ground. Next, place your shins on the swing. You should be in a push up / plank position with your shins on the swing. Keep your hands in place on the ground and your arms straight during the rock portion. Rock the swing forward and back two times. You will be pulling forward using your back / latissimus muscles and pushing backward using your shoulders. On the second forward rock of the swing, when your shoulders are beyond your hands, perform two push ups. Rock again and then perform another two push ups. You should feel this in your chest, triceps, shoulders, and core muscles. Repeat the swing rock with push ups for the desired number of repetitions.

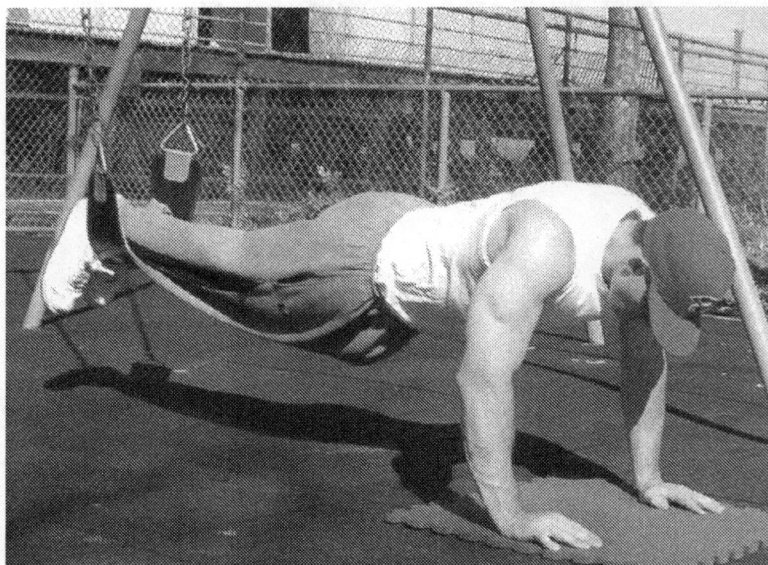

Advanced Full Body Workout 1

As you pull the swing forward, try not to allow your lower back to drop lower than the height of the swing.

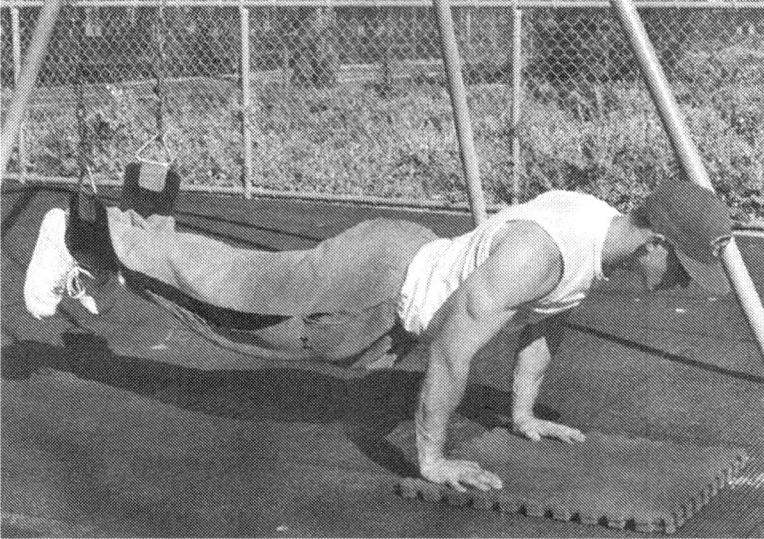

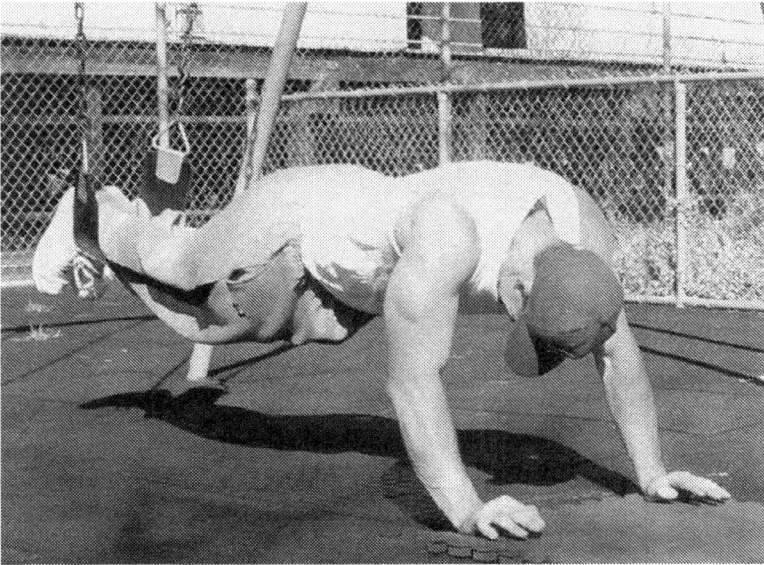

Swing Set Workouts

As you pull the swing forward, try not to allow your lower back to drop lower than the height of the swing.

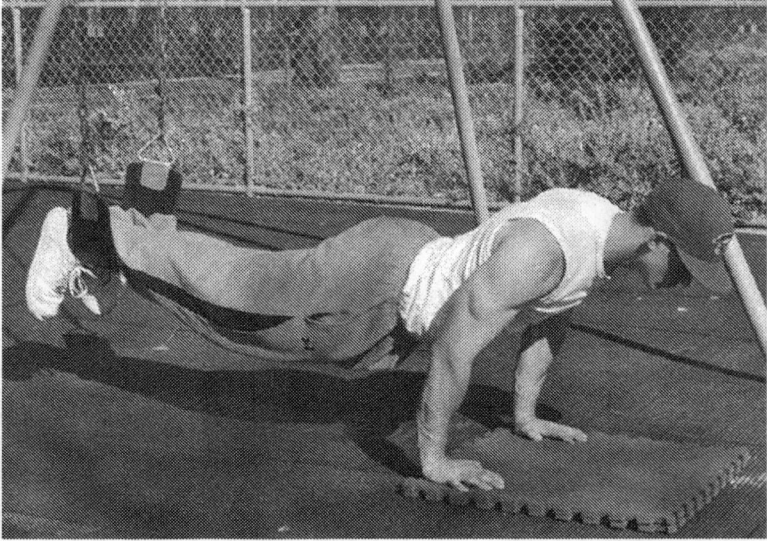

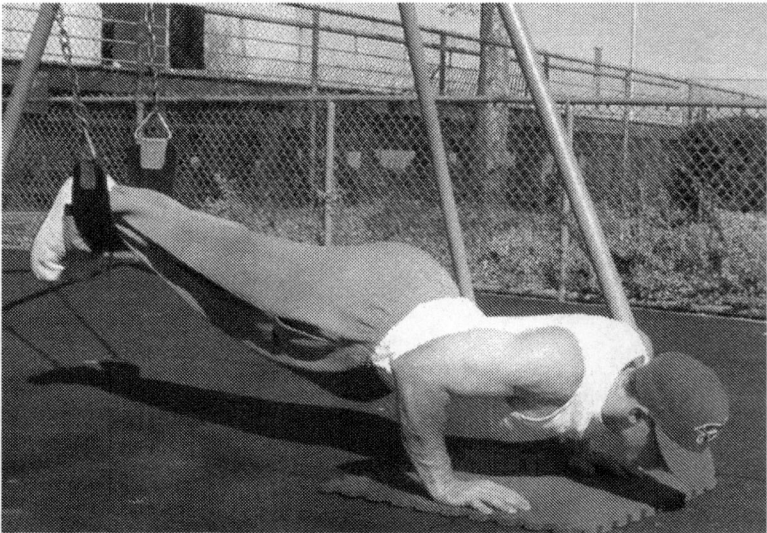

Always keep safety in mind!

Advanced Full Body Workout 1

Full Pike / Virtual Handstand with Shrug

Start with your back facing the swing. Place your hands on the ground. Next, place your shins on the swing. You should be in a push up / plank position with your shins on the swing. Next, pull your belly in so that you bend at the hips to form a full pike position, virtual handstand. Your hips will be directly above your head. Your legs and arms will remain straight. Your upper body will be in a virtual handstand. Once in the virtual handstand, shrug your shoulders so that your shoulders move toward your ears. Return to the straight push up / plank position and repeat the full pike and shrug for the desired number of repetitions. You should feel this in your core, chest, and shoulder muscles.

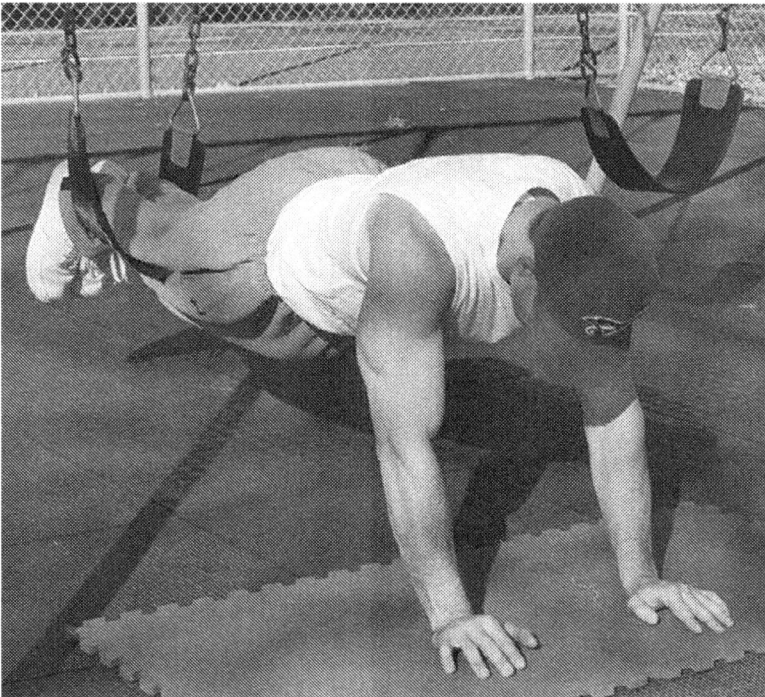

Swing Set Workouts

Only pull up to the full pike if you are strong enough to support your body weight upside down.

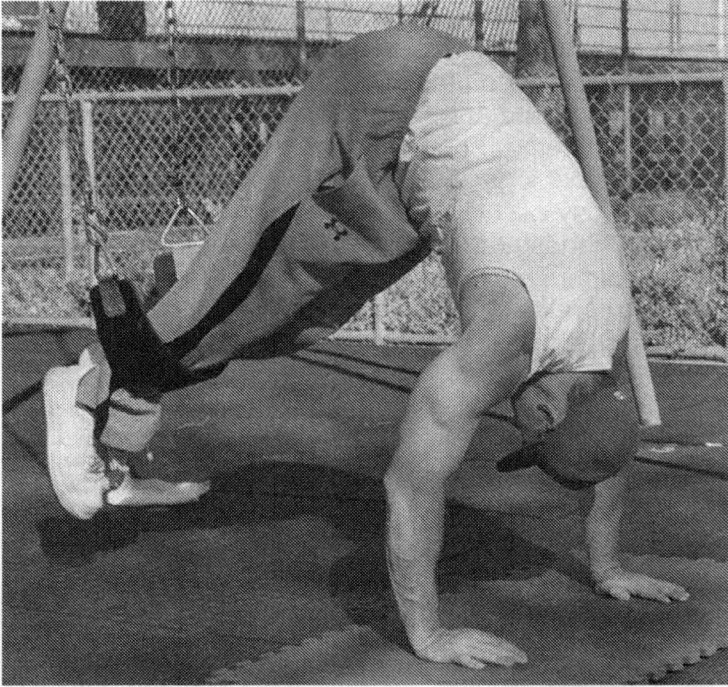

Always keep safety in mind!

Advanced Full Body Workout 1

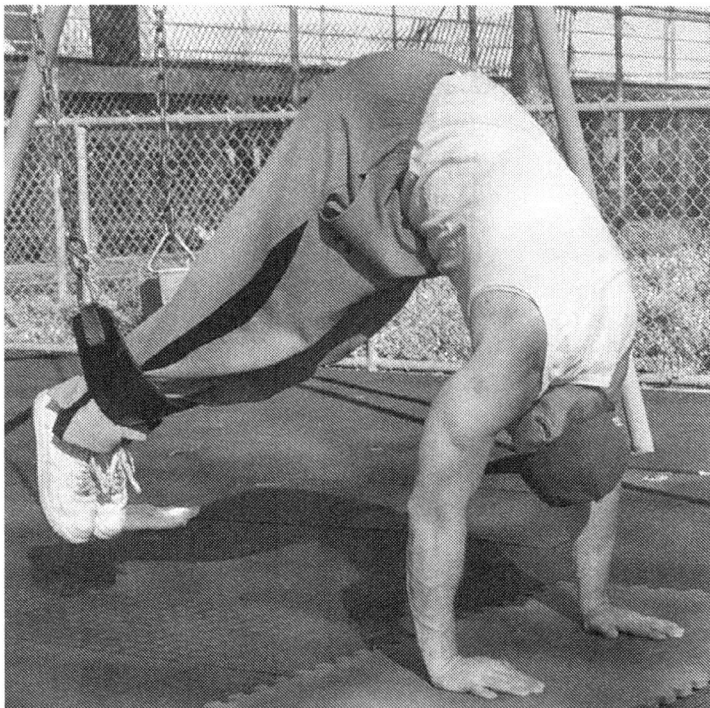

Single Leg Knee In - Tuck
Start with your back facing the swing. Place your hands on the ground. Next, place your shins on the swing. You should be in a push up / plank position with your shins on the swing. Next, lift your left leg 2-4 inches above the swing. Once the left leg is off the swing, pull your right knee toward your chest, bending at the hips to form a tuck position with that leg. Your hips will be slightly higher than your head and your thigh should be near your ribs. Your arms will remain straight. Return to the straight push / plank position and repeat the knee tuck for the desired number of repetitions. Perform this exercise with your left leg forming the tuck position. You should feel this in your core, chest, and shoulder muscles.

This exercise can be performed on your forearms to change the angle and muscle demand. It is also a great alternative if your wrists are sore.

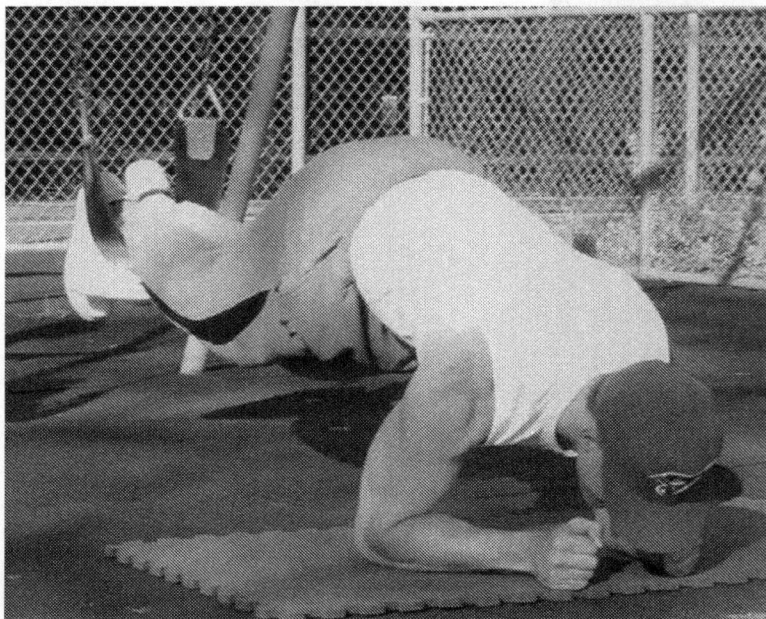

Advanced Full Body Workout 1

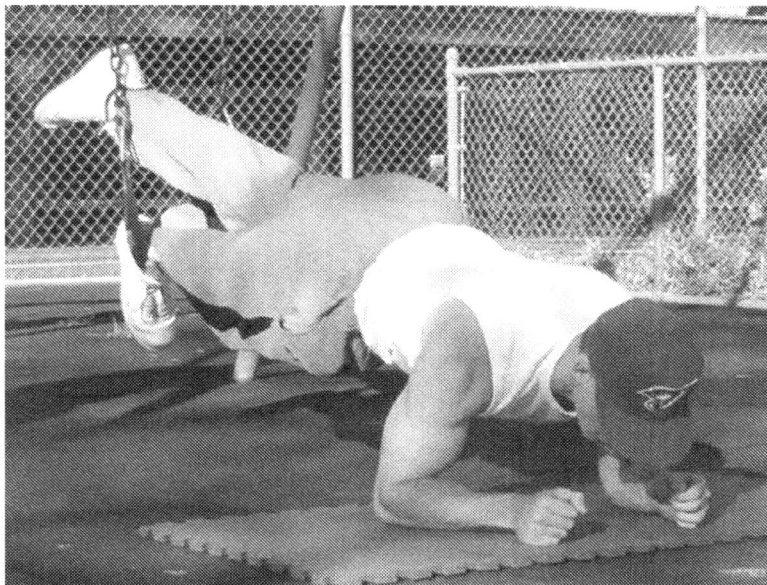

Swing Set Workouts

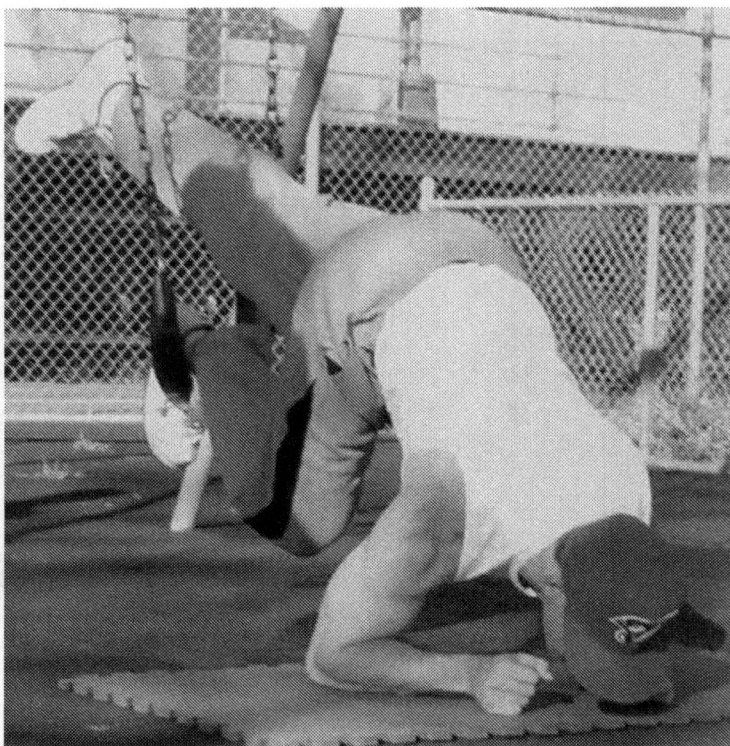

Always keep safety in mind!

Advanced Full Body Workout 1

Low Back Leg Lifts – Single Leg Lift

Start with your back facing the swing. Place your hands on the ground. Next, place your shins on the swing. You should be in a push up position with your shins on the swing. Next, lift your right leg off the swing 2-4 inches. Return that leg to the swing and repeat the lift for the desired number of repetitions. Your arms and body will remain straight throughout the exercise. Perform this exercise with your other leg for the desired number of repetitions. You should feel this in your core muscles.

This exercise can be performed on your forearms. It is a great alternative if your wrists are sore.

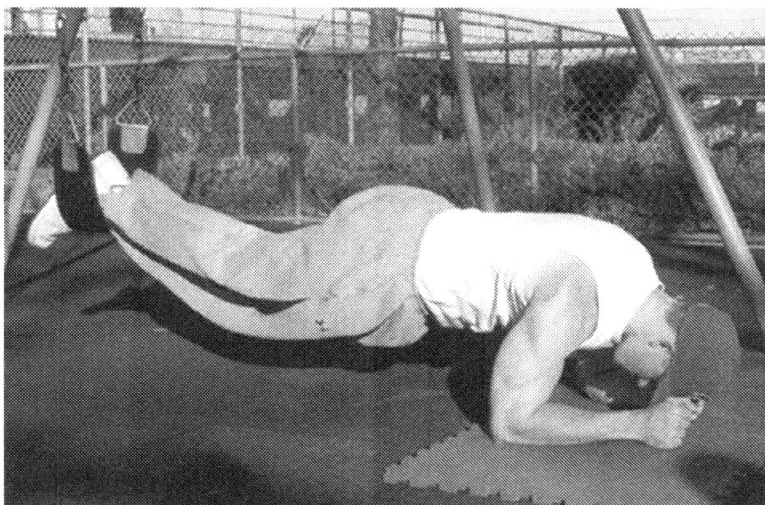

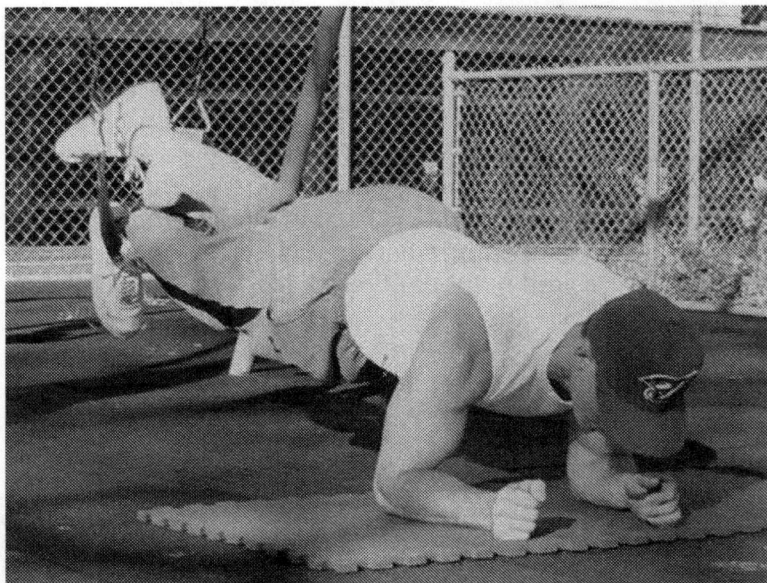

Always keep safety in mind!

Advanced Full Body Workout 2

If you enjoy a good challenge and working up a sweat, this workout is for you! There are 13 exercises in this workout.

Two to three sets per exercise are recommended and 10-15 repetitions per set are appropriate for this type of workout.

Swing Set Workouts

Always keep safety in mind!

Bulgarian Squat

Start with your back facing the swing. Lift your right foot up behind your body to place your right shin on the swing. Once you are balanced with your right shin on the swing, bend your left leg to perform a single leg squat. Make sure you keep your left knee in line with the hip and the toes on that side. Make sure you do not allow your knee to move forward, beyond your toes. Keep your chest up throughout the exercise.

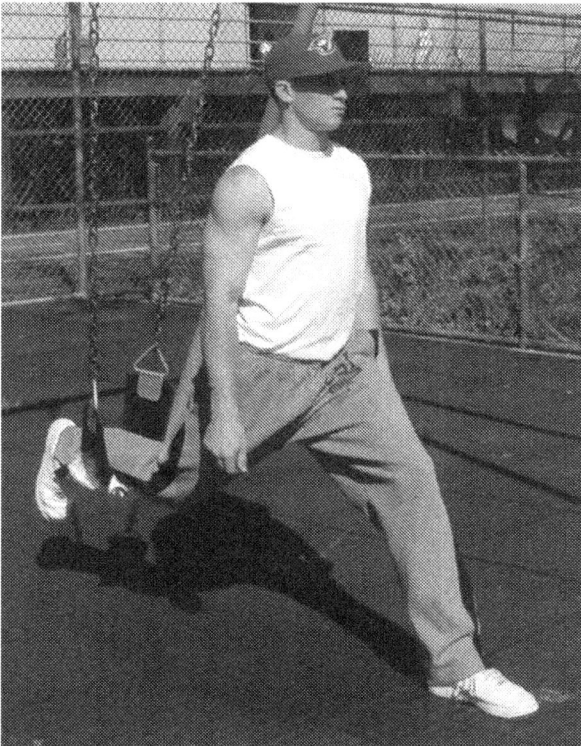

Swing Set Workouts

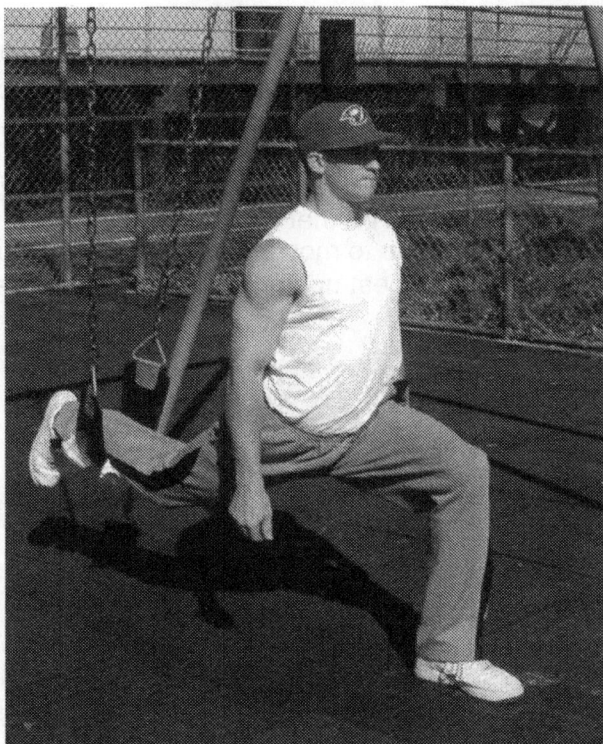

Always keep safety in mind!

Advanced Full Body Workout 2

Single Leg Swing Squat – Hold Swing

Start facing the swing. Grasp the outer portion of the swing with both hands and wrap fingers over the swing. Holding the swing securely, lean backward and walk your feet forward so that you are at approximately a 45 degree angle. Make sure your feet will not slide. Lift your right foot off the ground and hold the straight leg up in front of your body. Keep your chest up and bend your left knee to perform a single leg squat. Make sure you keep your left knee in line with your left hip and toes. Make sure you do not allow your knee to bend to far forward beyond your toes. Straighten and bend your knee for the desired number of repetitions. Perform this exercise for the same number of repetitions with your other leg.

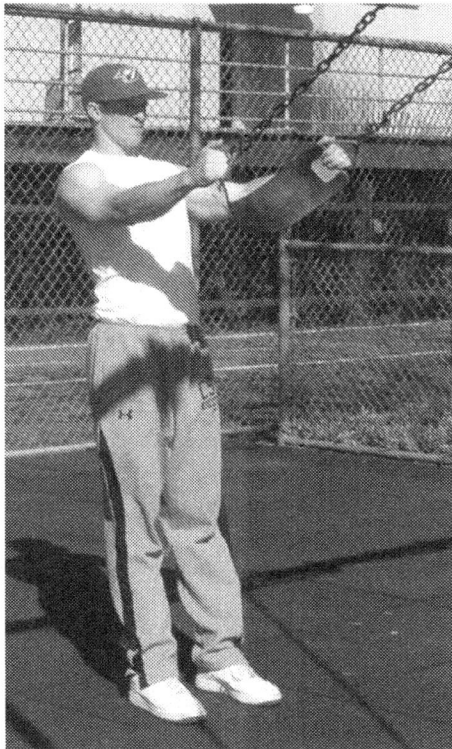

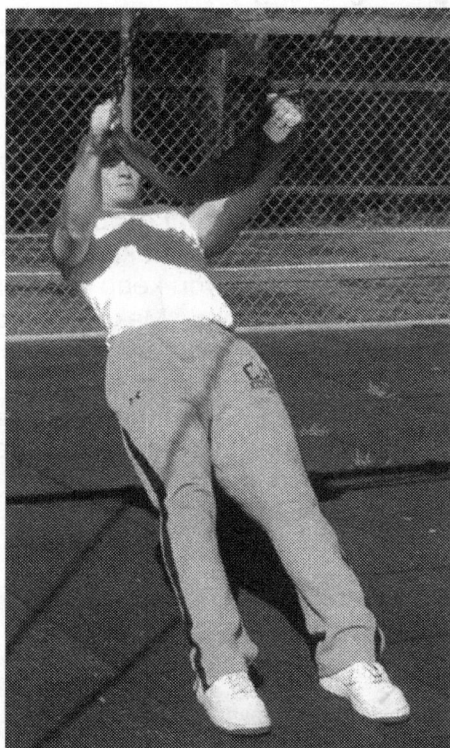

Always keep safety in mind!

Advanced Full Body Workout 2

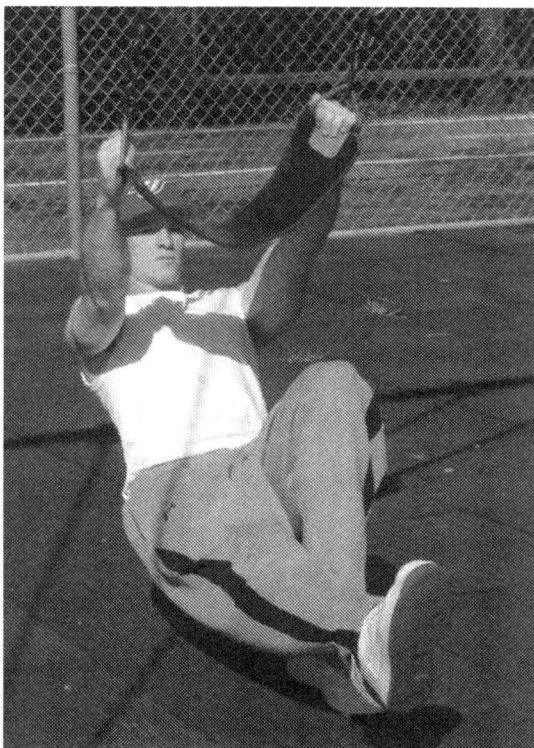

Lunge - Step Back

Start facing the swing. Grasp the outer portion of the swing with both hands and wrap fingers over the swing. Keeping your fingers wrapped around the bottom of the swing, step backward with your right leg and lower that knee toward the ground. Do not allow the knee or foot to touch the ground. Think of leaning back as you lunge. Lift off the ground using the quadriceps in the left leg and return to the starting position. Keep your chest up throughout the exercise. Make sure you keep your supporting knee in line with your hip and the toes on that side. Make sure you do not allow your knee to bend greater than a 90 degree angle.

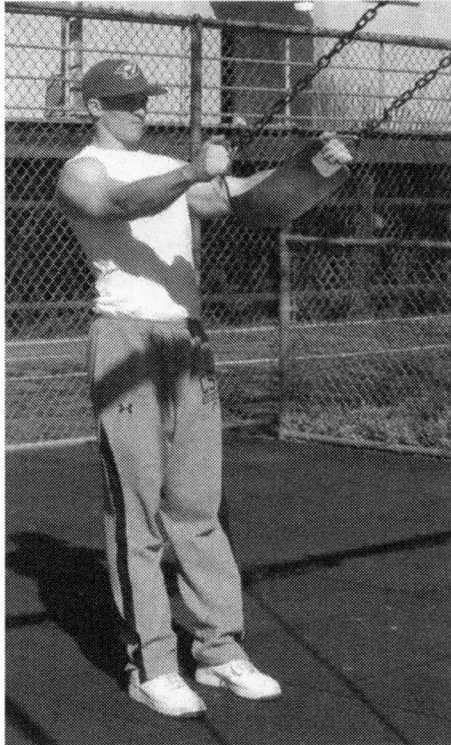

Always keep safety in mind!

Advanced Full Body Workout 2

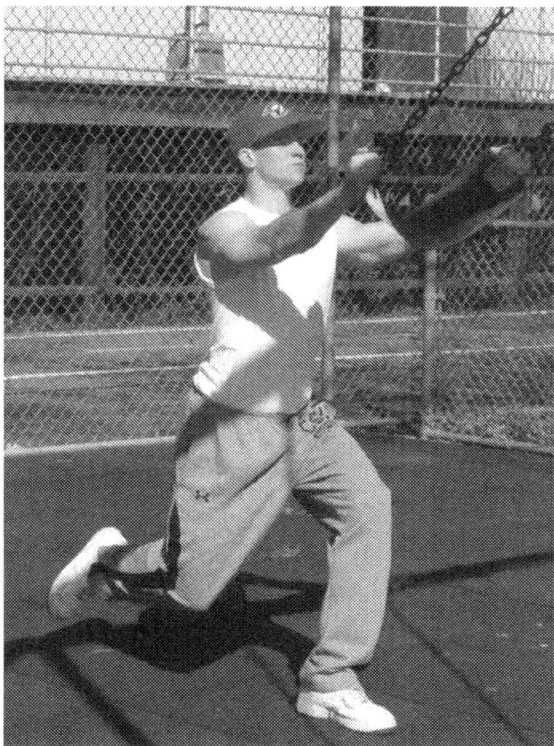

Swing Set Workouts

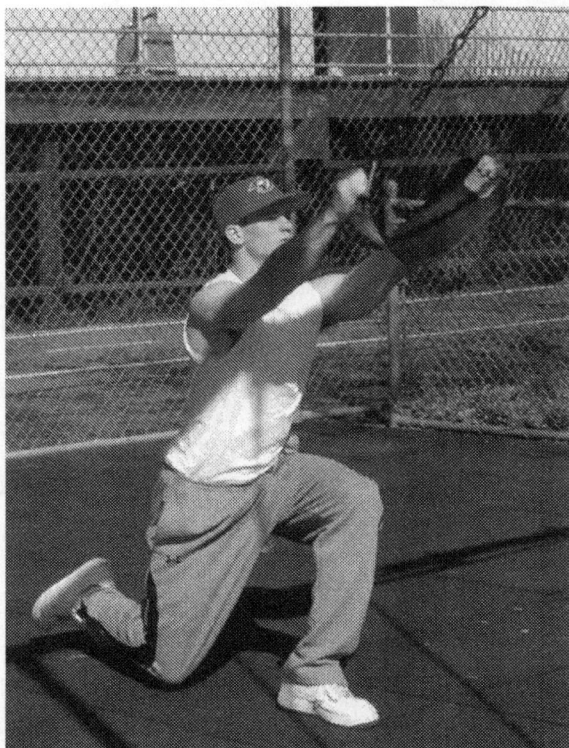

Always keep safety in mind!

Advanced Full Body Workout 2

Modified Pull Up – High

Grasp the outer portion of the swing with both hands and wrap fingers over the swing. Keeping your fingers wrapped around the bottom of the swing, lean backward and move your feet forward so that you are at a slight angle. Make sure your feet will not slide. Next, pull your chest in towards the swing. Keep your body straight throughout this exercise. You should feel this in your back and biceps.

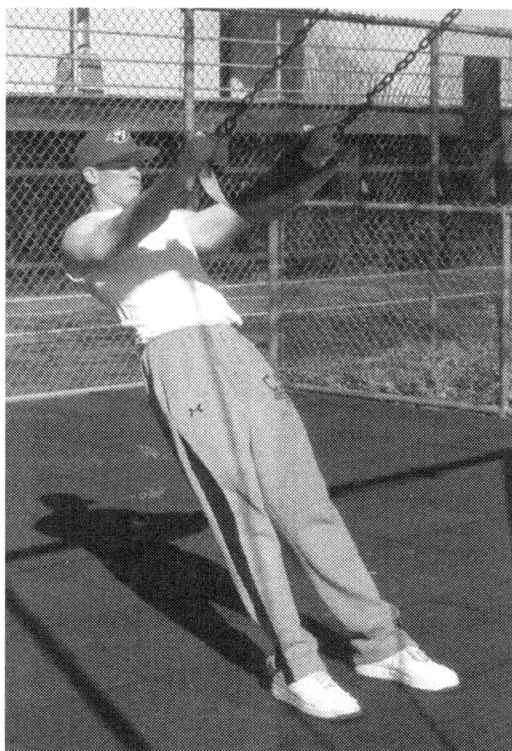

Swing Set Workouts

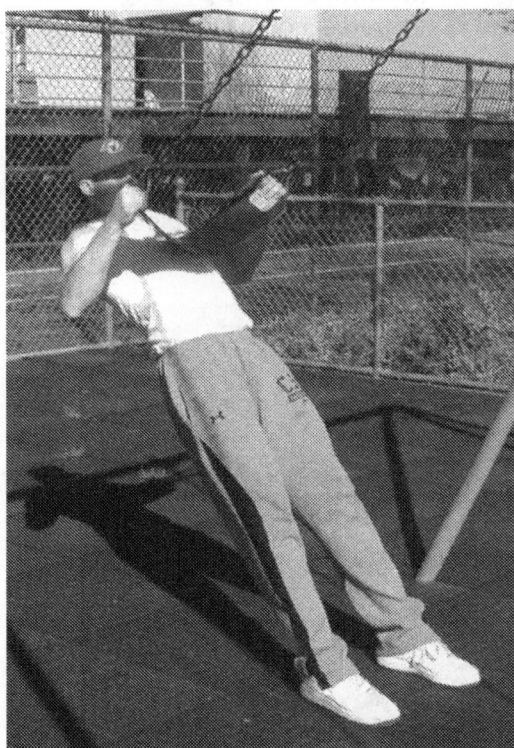

Always keep safety in mind!

Advanced Full Body Workout 2

Swing Protractions/ Shrugs (Swing)

Grasp the pouter portion of the swing with both hands. Keeping your fingers wrapped around the bottom of the swing, walk your feet backwards so that you are at an angle. Next, pull in your chest and raise your upper back toward the sky. The portion of your back between your shoulder blades will become rounded. Return to the push up position and press up again. It is a chest and shoulder motion. Your arms and legs remain straight. Repeat the protractions for the desired number of repetitions. You should feel this in your chest, triceps, and core muscles.

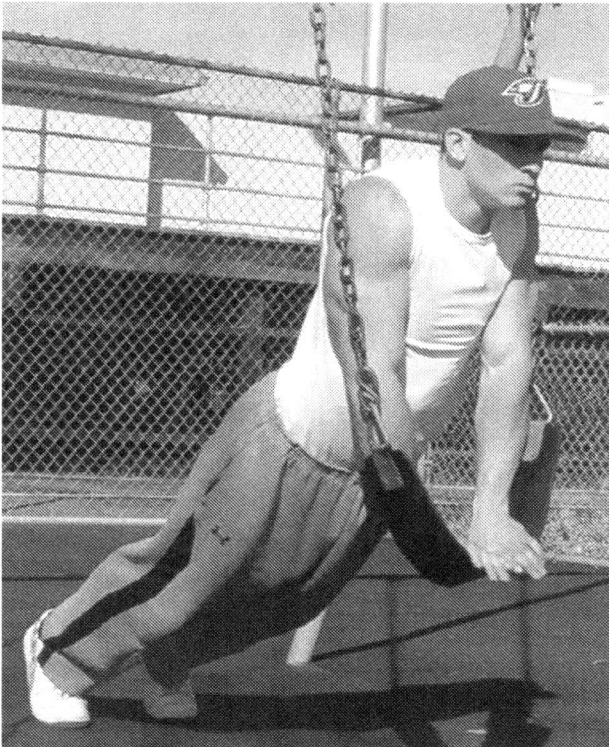

Swing Set Workouts

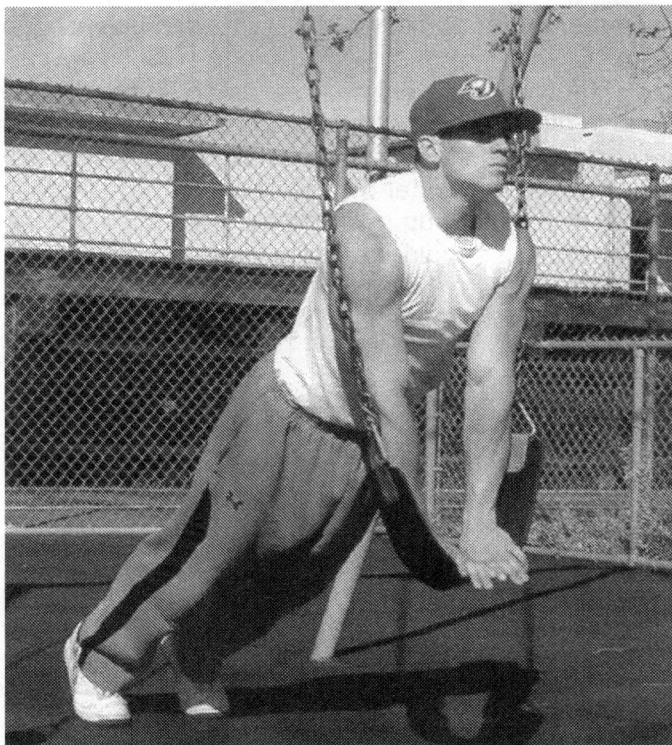

Always keep safety in mind!

Advanced Full Body Workout 2

Explosive Push Ups

Start with your back facing the swing. Place your hands on the ground. Next, place your shins on the swing. You should be in a push up / plank position with your shins on the swing. Once positioned, lower your chest and chin toward the ground and then in an explosive motion, push your body up into the air. If performed correctly, your hands will leave the ground for the brief moment, because you have jumped. Make sure you bend your elbows immediately upon contact with the ground. Keep your core muscles tight and do not allow your lower back to hang down. Repeat for the desired number of repetitions. You should feel this in your chest, triceps, and core muscles.

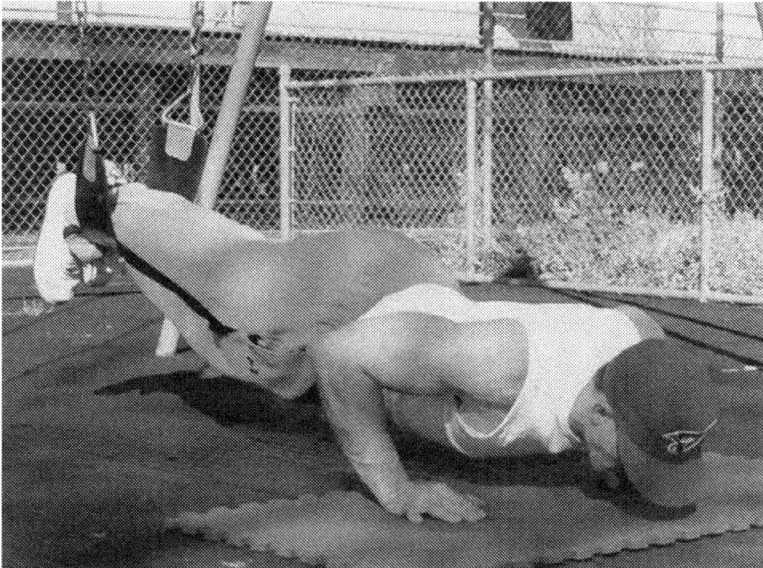

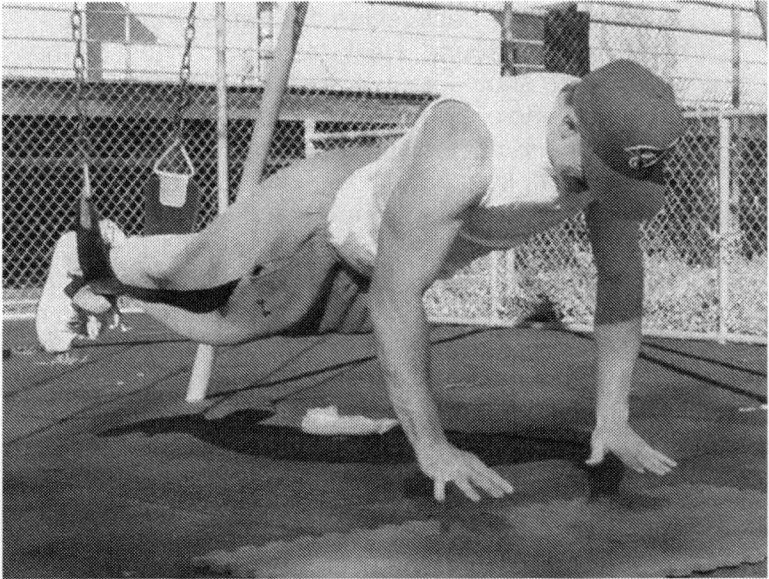

Make sure you bend your elbows immediately upon contact with the ground.

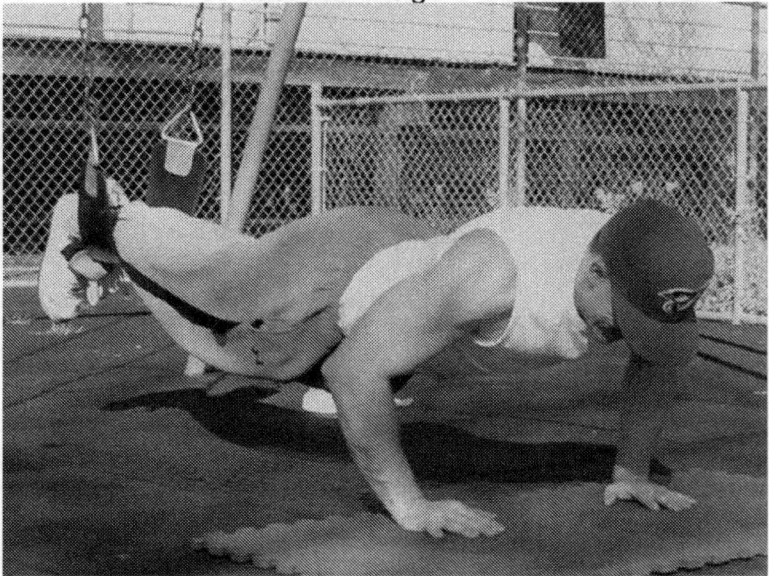

Always keep safety in mind!

Advanced Full Body Workout 2

Knee In Tuck

Start with your back facing the swing. Place your hands on the ground. Next, place your shins on the swing. You should be in a push up / plank position with your shins on the swing. Next, pull your knees toward your chest, bending at the hips to form a tuck position. Your hips will be slightly higher than your head and your thighs should be touching your ribs. Your arms will remain straight. Return to the straight push / plank position and repeat the knee tuck for the desired number of repetitions. You should feel this in your core, chest, and shoulder muscles.

This exercise can be performed on your forearms to change the angle and muscle demand. It is also a great alternative if your wrists are sore.

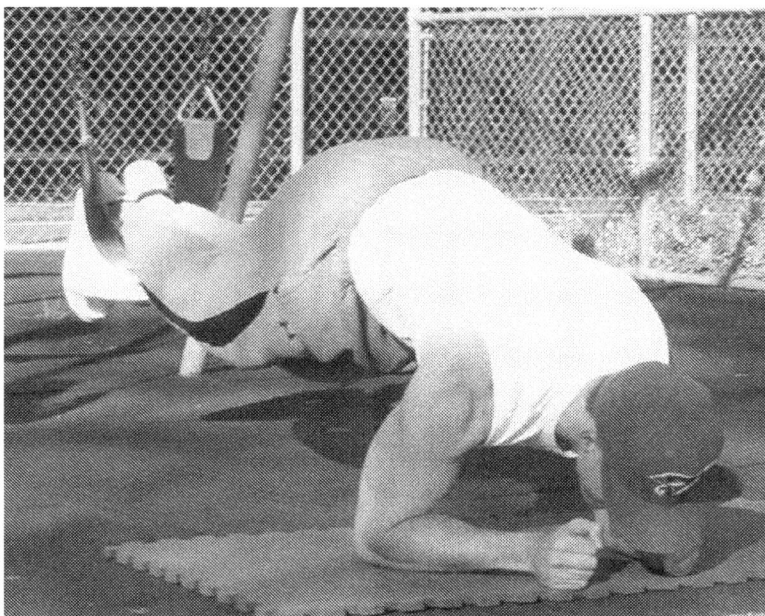

Swing Set Workouts

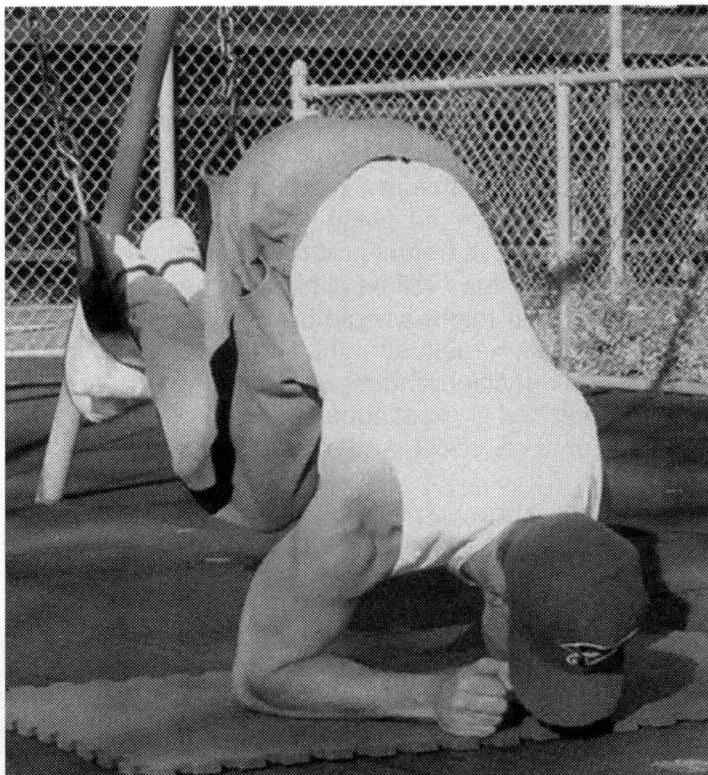

Always keep safety in mind!

Advanced Full Body Workout 2

Single Leg Knee In - Tuck
Start with your back facing the swing. Place your hands on the ground. Next, place your shins on the swing. You should be in a push up / plank position with your shins on the swing. Next, lift your left leg 2-4 inches above the swing. Once the left leg is off the swing, pull your right knee toward your chest, bending at the hips to form a tuck position with that leg. Your hips will be slightly higher than your head and your thigh should be near your ribs. Your arms will remain straight. Return to the straight push / plank position and repeat the knee tuck for the desired number of repetitions. Perform this exercise with your left leg forming the tuck position. You should feel this in your core, chest, and shoulder muscles.

This exercise can be performed on your forearms to change the angle and muscle demand. It is also a great alternative if your wrists are sore.

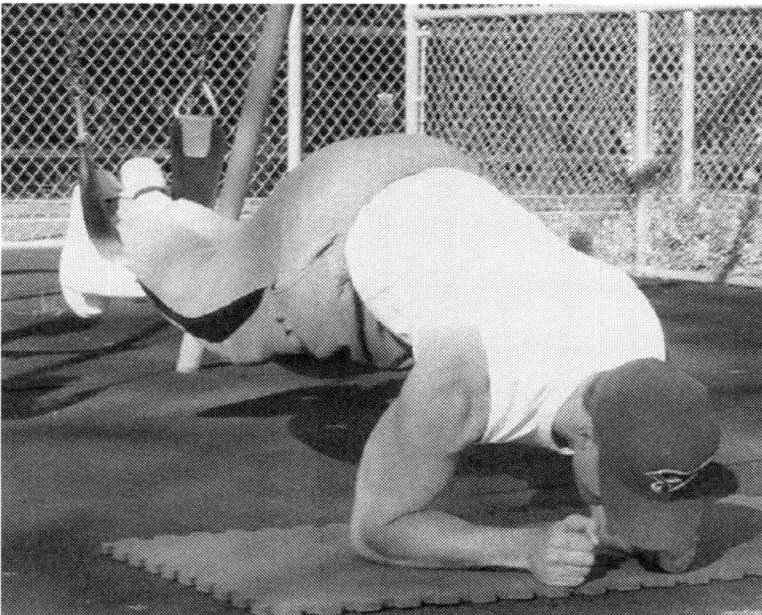

Swing Set Workouts

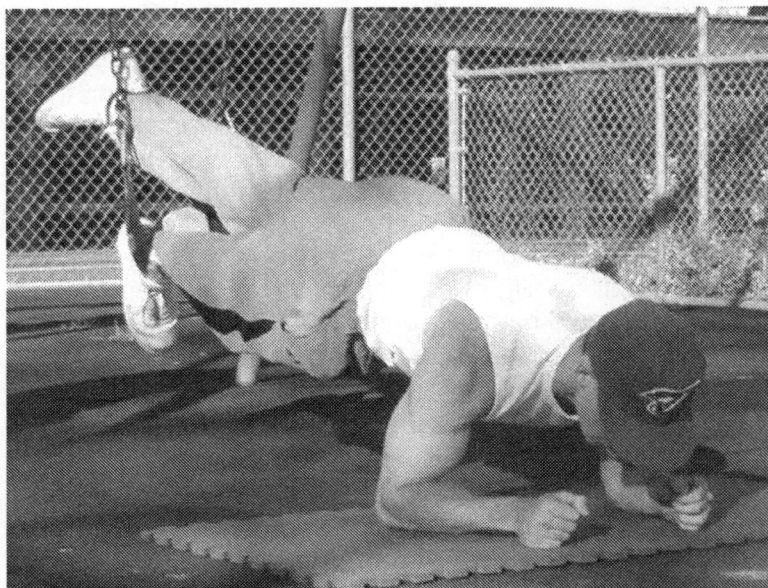

Always keep safety in mind!

Advanced Full Body Workout 2

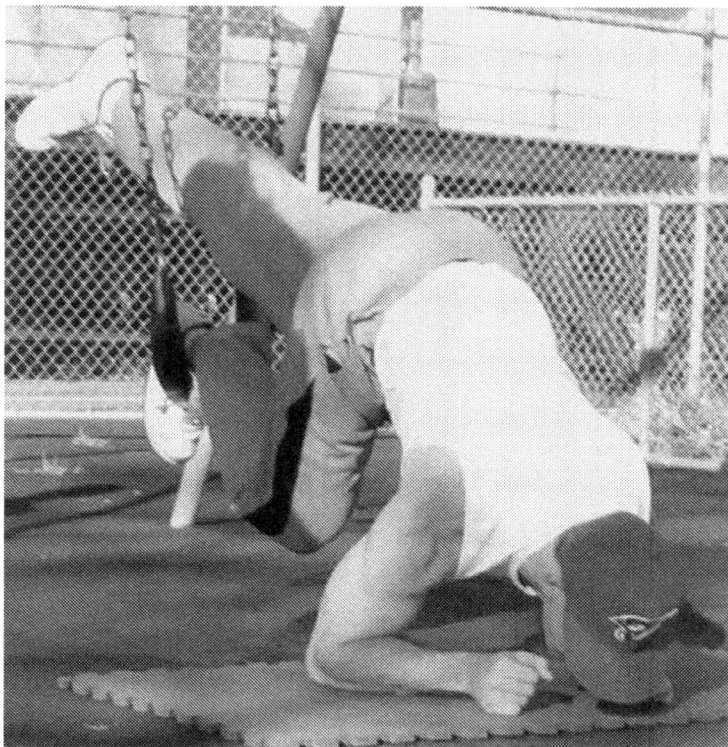

Legs and Shoulders

This is an advanced workout. It is for people who train each body area one time per week using split routines. Your core muscles will be also become involved with some of the exercises included in this workout.

Three sets per exercise are recommended and 10-15 repetitions per set are appropriate for this type of workout. Perform no more than four sets per exercise.

Swing Set Workouts

Always keep safety in mind!

Legs and Shoulders

Squat – Hold Swing (Lean Back)

Start facing the swing. Grasp the outer portion of the swing with both hands and wrap fingers over the swing. (Other option is to grasp the lowest portion of the chains.) Holding the swing securely, lean backward and walk your feet forward so that you are at approximately a 45 degree angle. Make sure your feet will not slide. Keep your chest up and bend both knees to perform a squat. Make sure your knees remain in line with your hips. Do not allow your knees to fall toward each other. Make sure your knees do not go forward beyond your toes. Straighten and bend your knees for the desired number of repetitions.

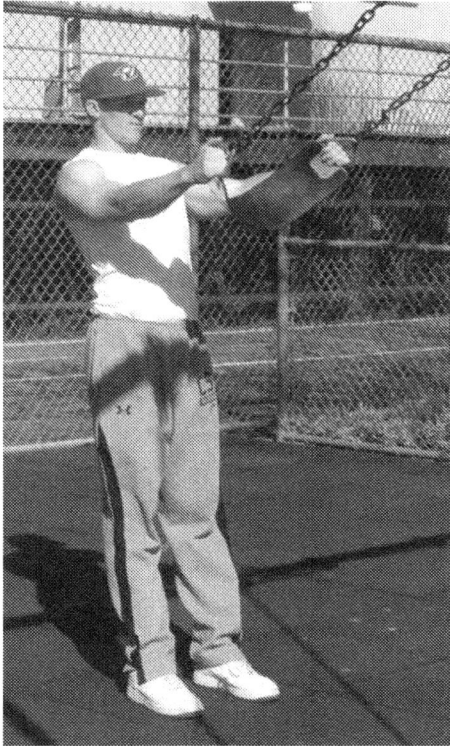

Swing Set Workouts

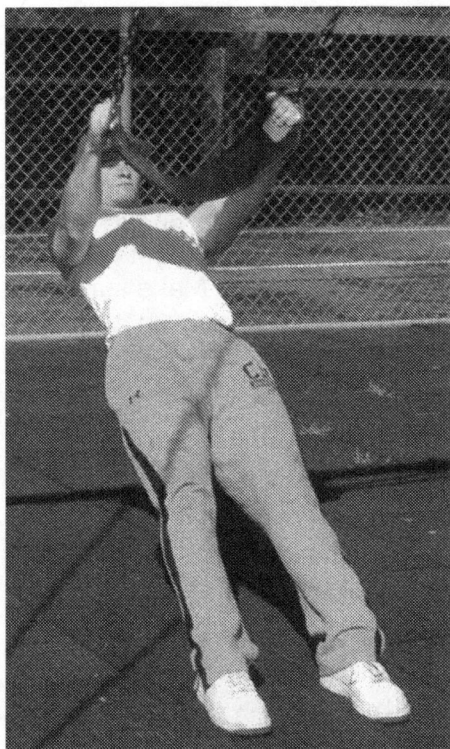

Always keep safety in mind!

Legs and Shoulders

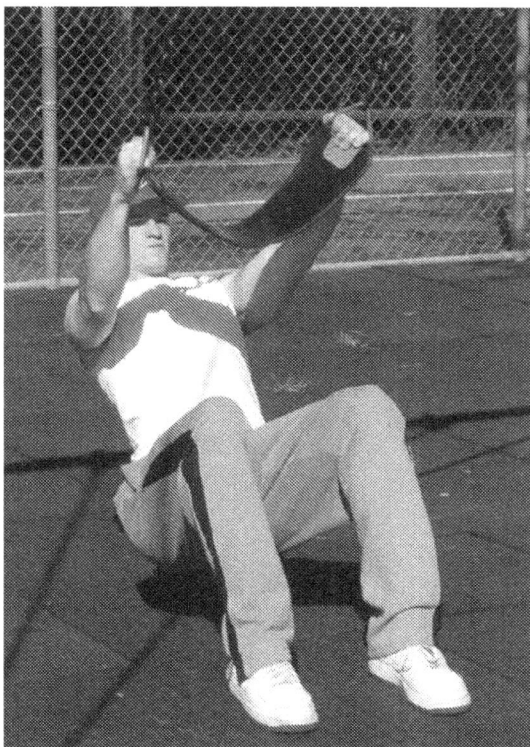

Swing Set Workouts

Single Leg Swing Squat – Hold Swing
Start facing the swing. Grasp the outer portion of the swing with both hands and wrap fingers over the swing. Holding the swing securely, lean backward and walk your feet forward so that you are at approximately a 45 degree angle. Make sure your feet will not slide. Lift your right foot off the ground and hold the straight leg up in front of your body. Keep your chest up and bend your left knee to perform a single leg squat. Make sure you keep your left knee in line with your left hip and toes. Make sure you do not allow your knee to bend to far forward beyond your toes. Straighten and bend your knee for the desired number of repetitions. Perform this exercise for the same number of repetitions with your other leg.

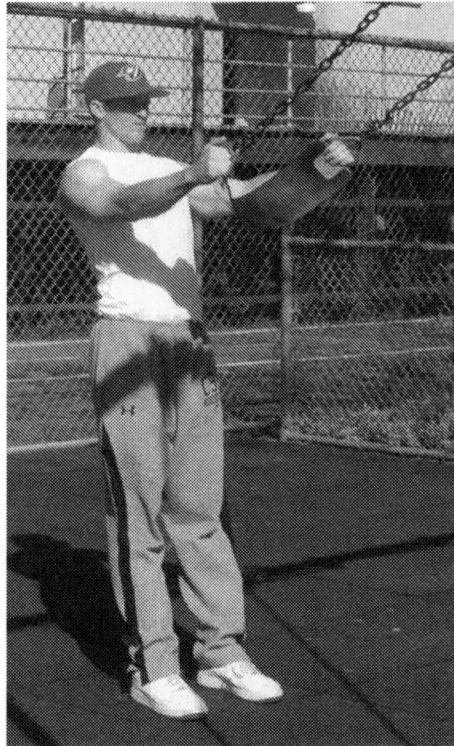

Always keep safety in mind!

Legs and Shoulders

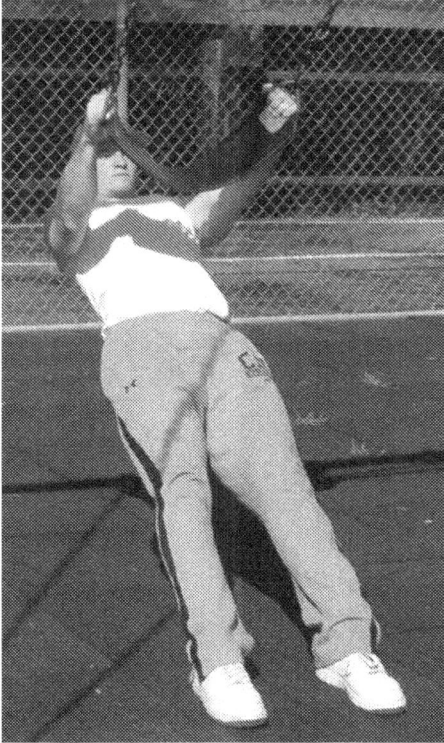

Swing Set Workouts

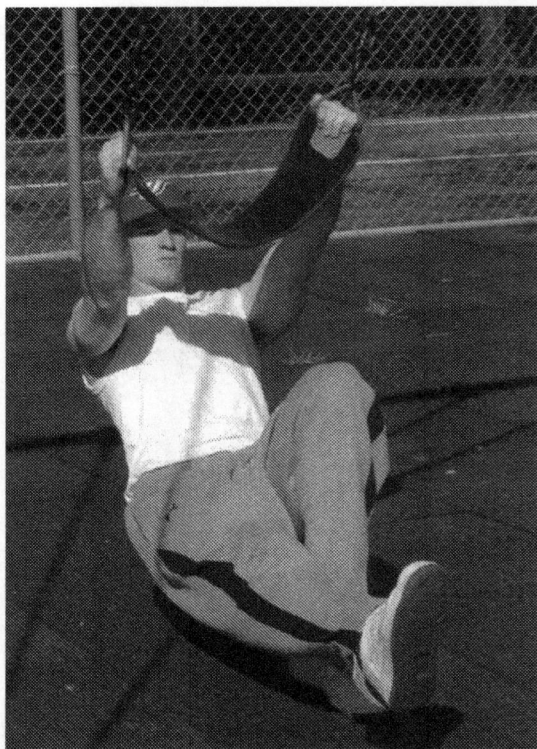

Always keep safety in mind!

Legs and Shoulders

Lunge - Step Back

Start facing the swing. Grasp the outer portion of the swing with both hands and wrap fingers over the swing. Keeping your fingers wrapped around the bottom of the swing, step backward with your right leg and lower that knee toward the ground. Do not allow the knee or foot to touch the ground. Think of leaning back as you lunge. Lift off the ground using the quadriceps in the left leg and return to the starting position. Keep your chest up throughout the exercise. Make sure you keep your supporting knee in line with your hip and the toes on that side. Make sure you do not allow your knee to bend greater than a 90 degree angle.

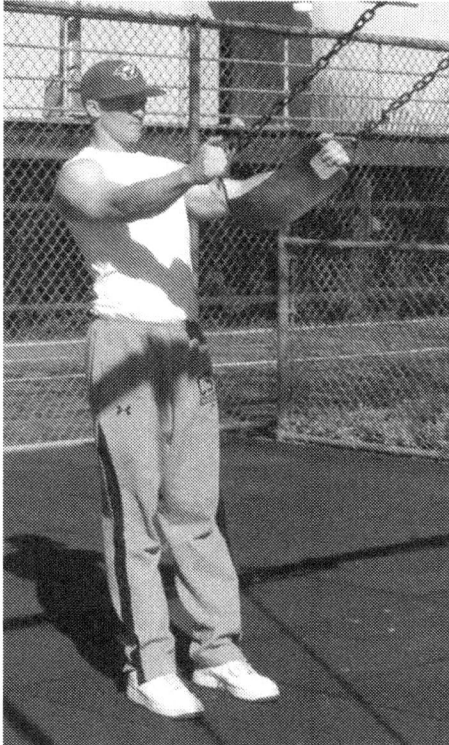

Swing Set Workouts

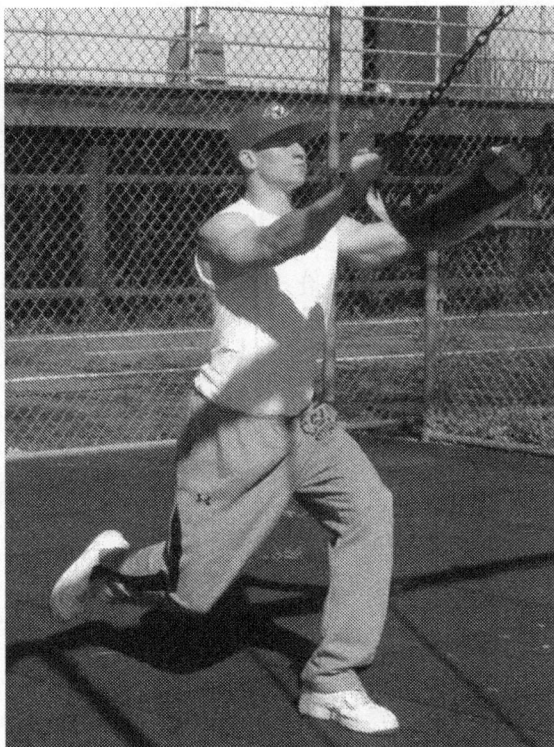

Always keep safety in mind!

Legs and Shoulders

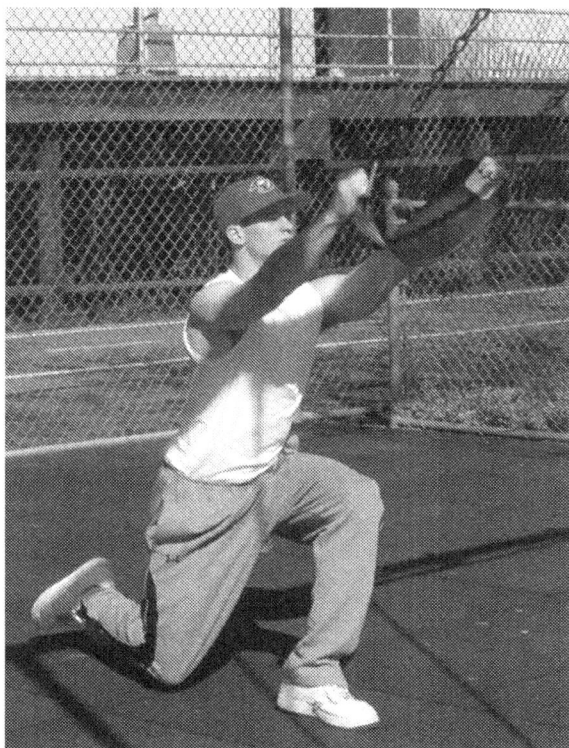

Calf Raise

Start facing the swing. Grasp the center of the swing with both hands. Keeping your fingers wrapped around the bottom of the swing, walk your feet backwards so that you are at an angle. Once in position, lift your heels off the ground. Return to the starting position. Continue to lift your heels for the desired number of repetitions. Keep your chest up and your body straight throughout this exercise.

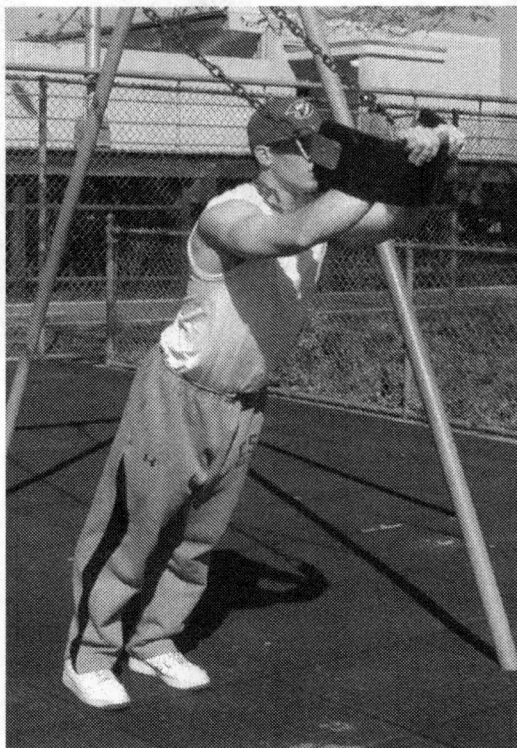

Always keep safety in mind!

Legs and Shoulders

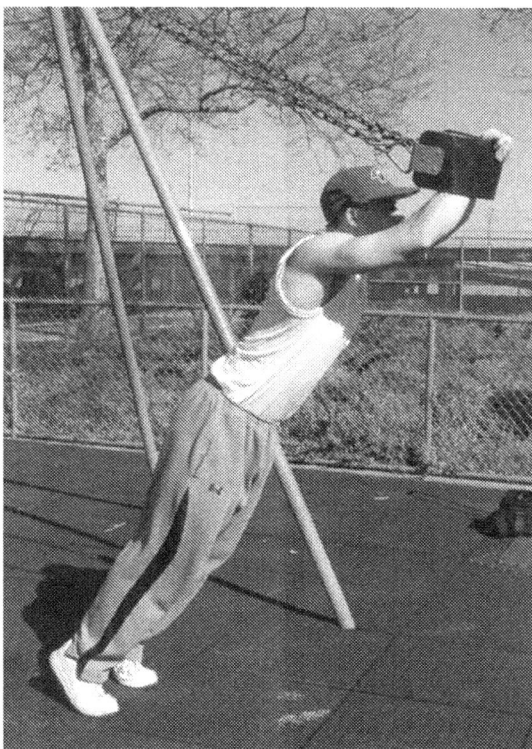

Swing Rocks / Pulls in Push Up Position

Start with your back facing the swing. Place your hands on the ground. Next, place your shins in the swing. You should be in a push up / plank position with your shins on the swing. Keep your hands in place in place on the ground and your arms straight throughout the exercise. Rock the swing forward and back. You will be pulling forward using your back / latissimus muscles and pushing backward using your shoulders. You should feel this in your chest, triceps, and shoulders, and core muscles. Repeat the swing rocks for the desired number of repetitions.

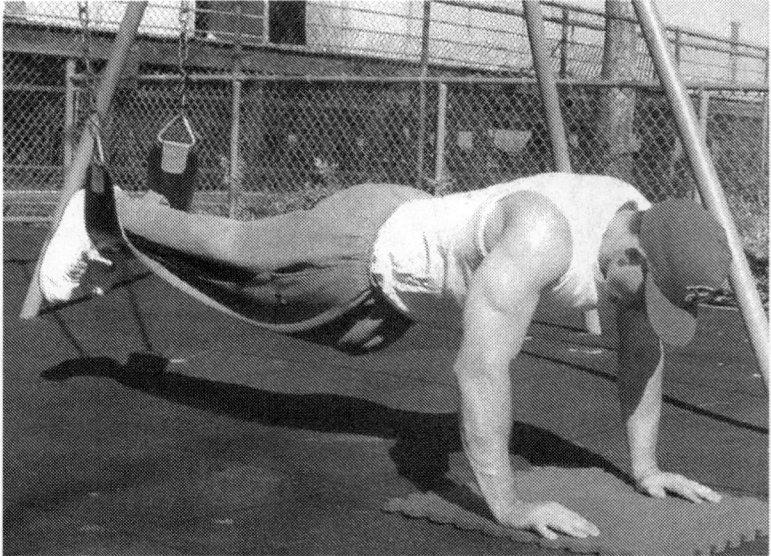

Legs and Shoulders

As you pull the swing forward, try not to allow your lower back t drop lower than the height of the swing.

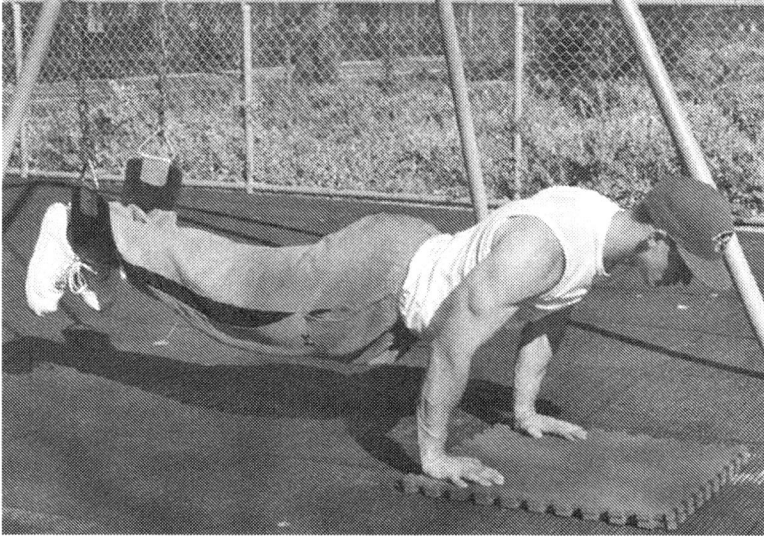

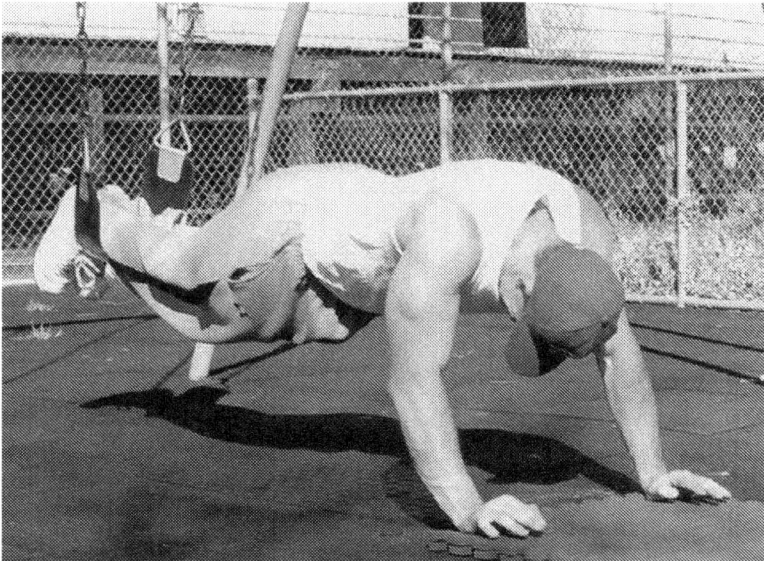

Swing Set Workouts

Swing Rocks / Pulls with Push Up

Start with your back facing the swing. Place your hands on the ground. Next, place your shins on the swing. You should be in a push up / plank position with your shins on the swing. Keep your hands in place on the ground and your arms straight during the rock portion. Rock the swing forward and back two times. You will be pulling forward using your back / latissimus muscles and pushing backward using your shoulders. On the second forward rock of the swing, when your shoulders are beyond your hands, perform two push ups. Rock again and then perform another two push ups. You should feel this in your chest, triceps, shoulders, and core muscles. Repeat the swing rock with push ups for the desired number of repetitions.

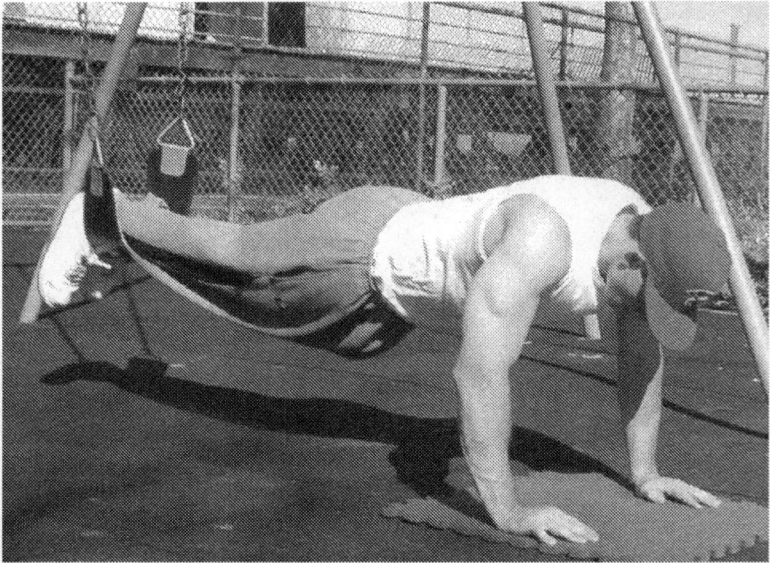

Always keep safety in mind!

Legs and Shoulders

As you pull the swing forward, try not to allow your lower back t drop lower than the height of the swing.

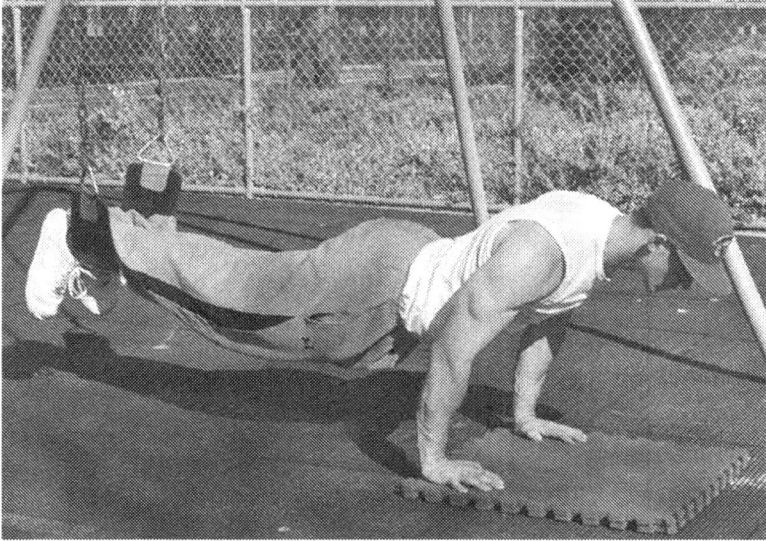

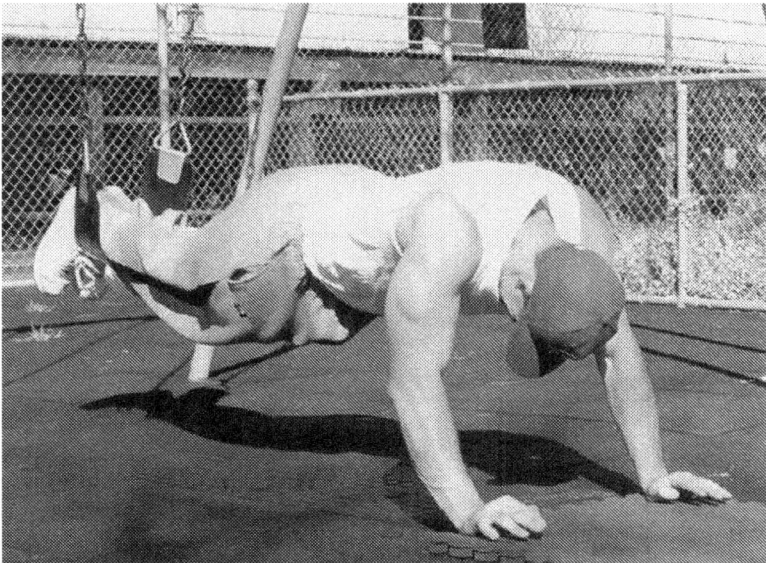

Swing Set Workouts

Full Pike / Virtual Handstand with Shrug

Start with your back facing the swing. Place your hands on the ground. Next, place your shins on the swing. You should be in a push up / plank position with your shins on the swing. Next, pull your belly in so that you bend at the hips to form a full pike position, virtual handstand. Your hips will be directly above your head. Your legs and arms will remain straight. Your upper body will be in a virtual handstand. Once in the virtual handstand, shrug your shoulders so that your shoulders move toward your ears. Return to the straight push up / plank position and repeat the full pike and shrug for the desired number of repetitions. You should feel this in your core, chest, and shoulder muscles.

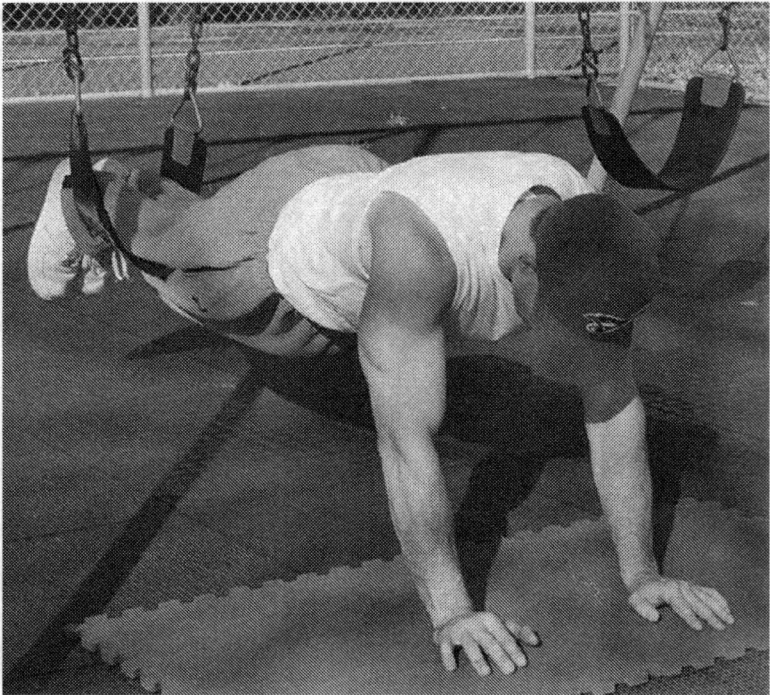

Always keep safety in mind!

Legs and Shoulders

Only pull up to the full pike if you are strong enough to support your body weight upside down.

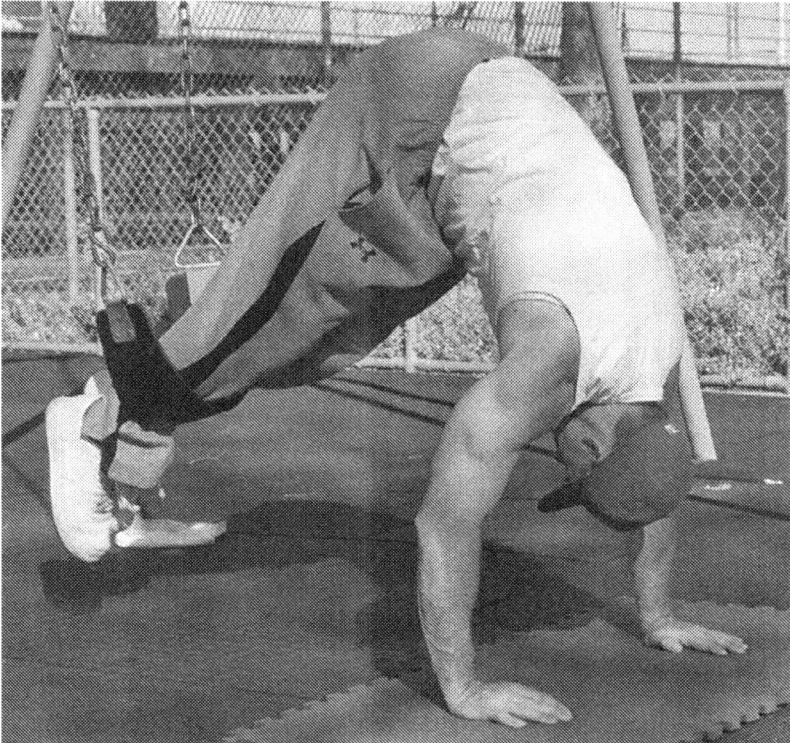

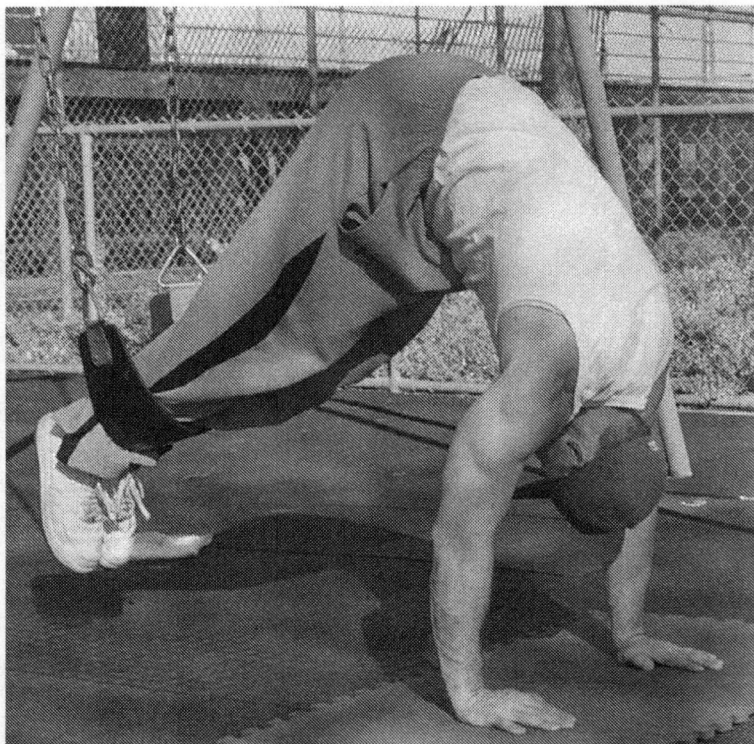

Always keep safety in mind!

Legs and Shoulders

As you pull the swing forward, try not to allow your lower back t drop lower than the height of the swing.

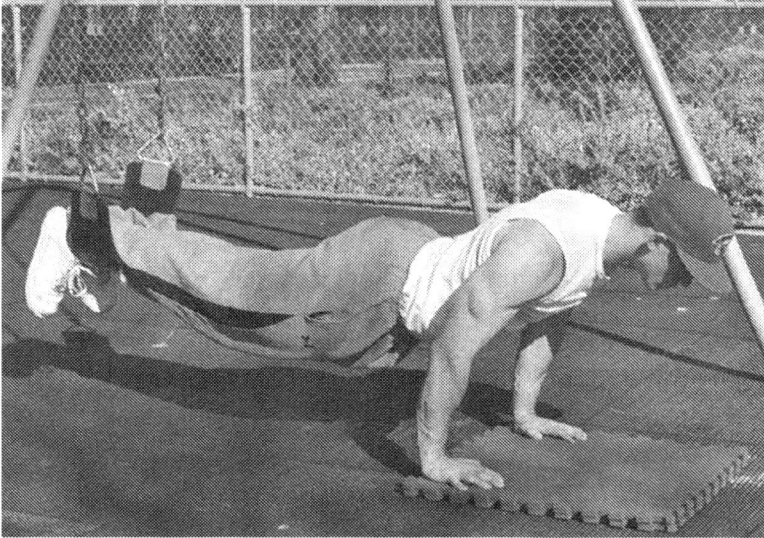

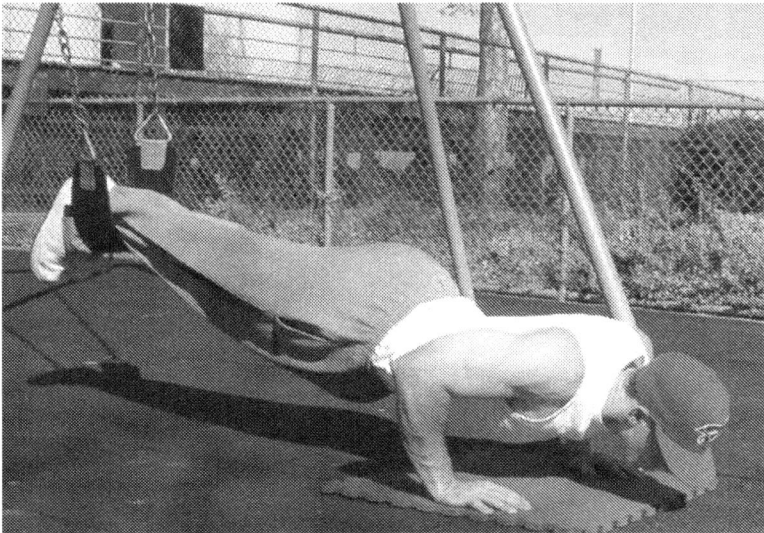

Swing Set Workouts

Pike / Virtual Handstand Push Up

Start with your back facing the swing. Place your hands on the ground. Next, place your shins on the swing. You should be in a push up / plank position with your shins on the swing. Next, pull your belly in so that you bend at the hips to form a full pike position, virtual handstand. Your hips will be directly above your head. Once in the virtual handstand, bend your elbows so that your head moves towards the ground. Do not allow your head to touch the ground! Your legs will remain straight. Your upper body will be in a virtual handstand during these push ups. Return to the virtual handstand and then to the straight push up / plank position. Repeat the handstand pushup for the desired number of repetitions. You should feel this in your shoulders and core muscles.

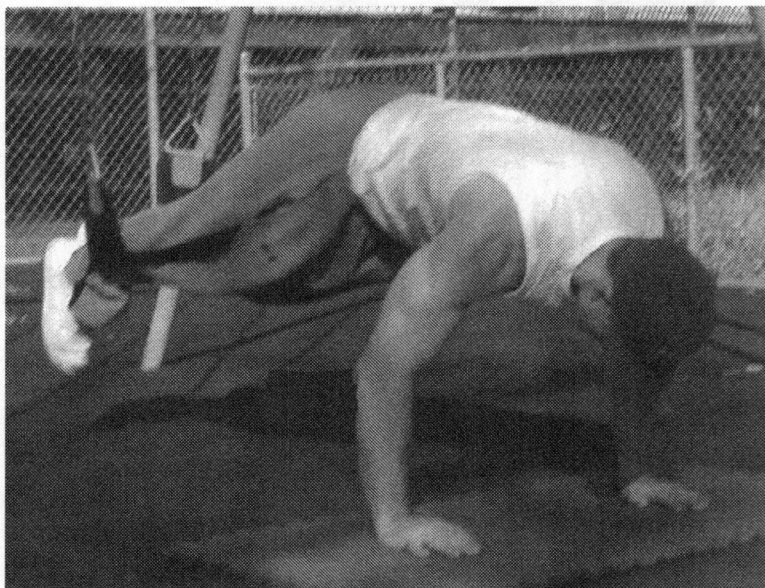

Always keep safety in mind!

Legs and Shoulders

Do not allow your head or face to contact the ground. Only perform this exercise of you are strong enough to support yourself upside down.

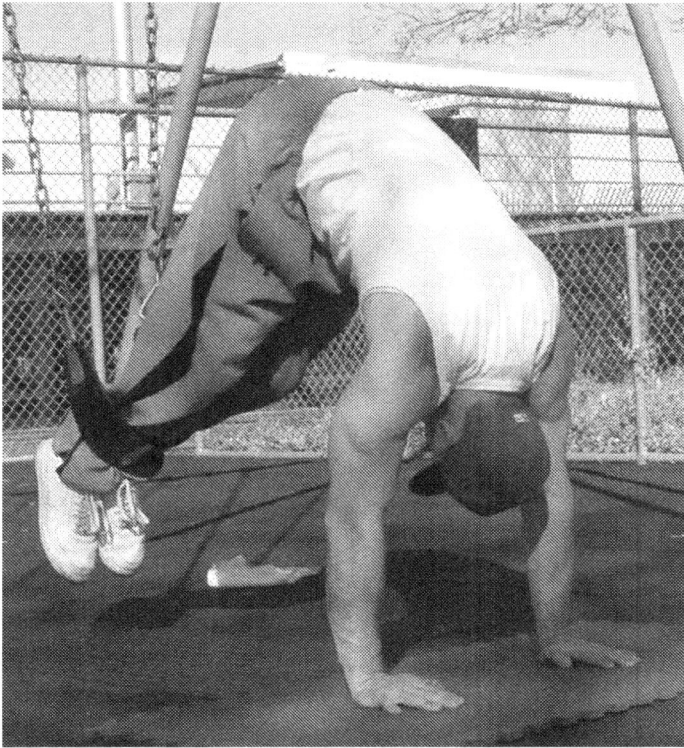

Swing Set Workouts

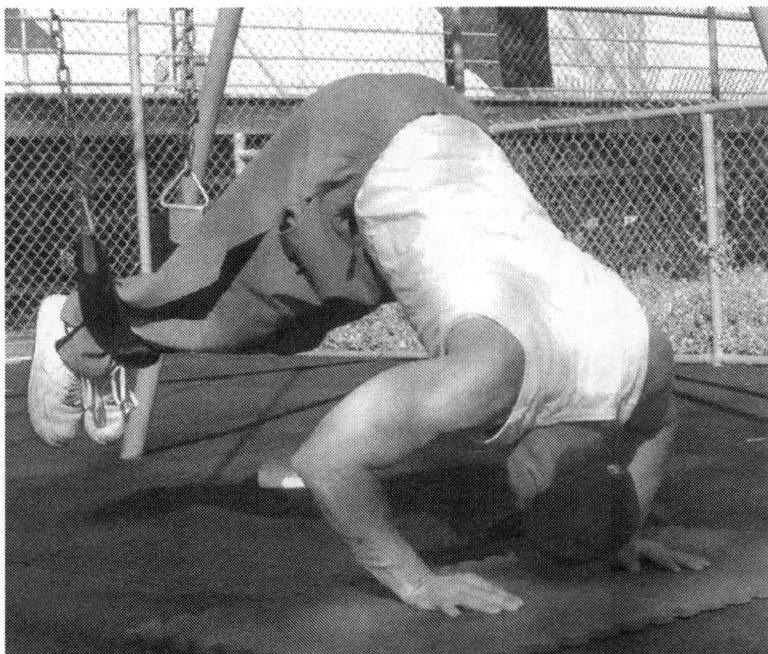

Always keep safety in mind!

Legs and Shoulders

Chest and Arms

This is an advanced workout. It is for people who train each body area one time per week using split routines. Your core muscles will be also become involved with some of the exercises included in this workout

Three sets per exercise are recommended and 10-15 repetitions per set are appropriate for this type of workout. Perform no more than four sets per exercise.

Swing Set Workouts

Always keep safety in mind!

Chest and Arms

Swing Push Ups – Shins on Swing

Start with your back facing the swing. Place your hands on the ground. Next, place your shins on the swing. You should be in a push up position with your shins on the swing. Once positioned, lower your chest and chin near the ground and then push back up. Keep your core muscles tight and do not allow your lower back to hang down. Repeat for the desired number of repetitions. You should feel this in your chest, triceps, and core muscles.

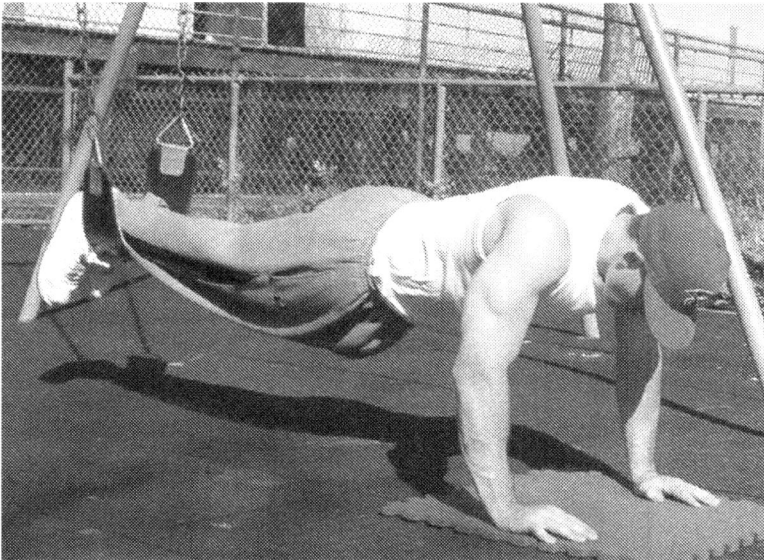

Swing Set Workouts

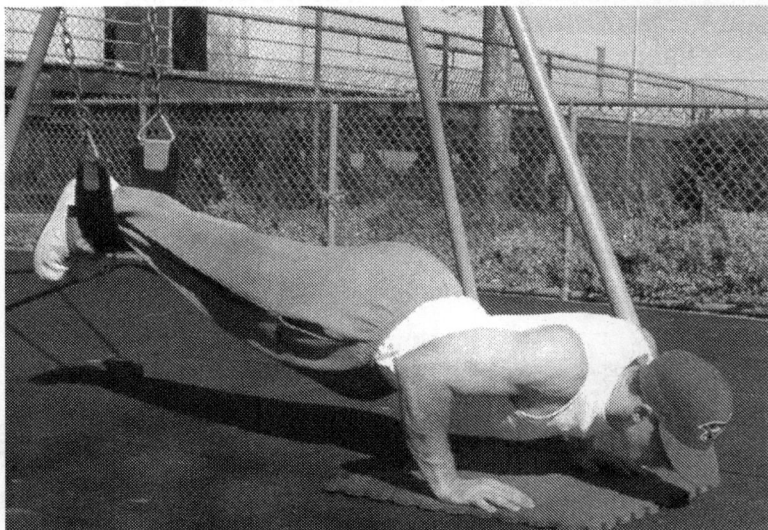

Always keep safety in mind!

Chest and Arms

Swing Rocks / Pulls with Push Up

Start with your back facing the swing. Place your hands on the ground. Next, place your shins on the swing. You should be in a push up / plank position with your shins on the swing. Keep your hands in place on the ground and your arms straight during the rock portion. Rock the swing forward and back two times. You will be pulling forward using your back / latissimus muscles and pushing backward using your shoulders. On the second forward rock of the swing, when your shoulders are beyond your hands, perform two push ups. Rock again and then perform another two push ups. You should feel this in your chest, triceps, shoulders, and core muscles. Repeat the swing rock with push ups for the desired number of repetitions.

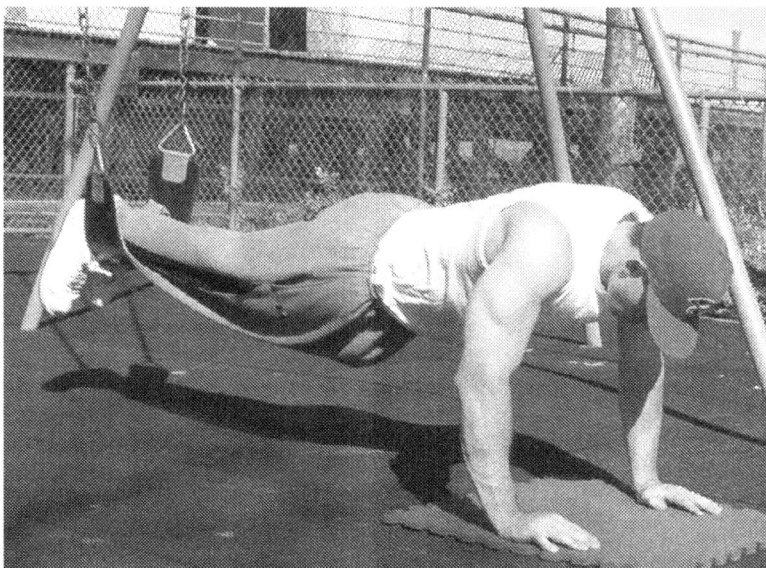

Swing Set Workouts

As you pull the swing forward, try not to allow your lower back t drop lower than the height of the swing.

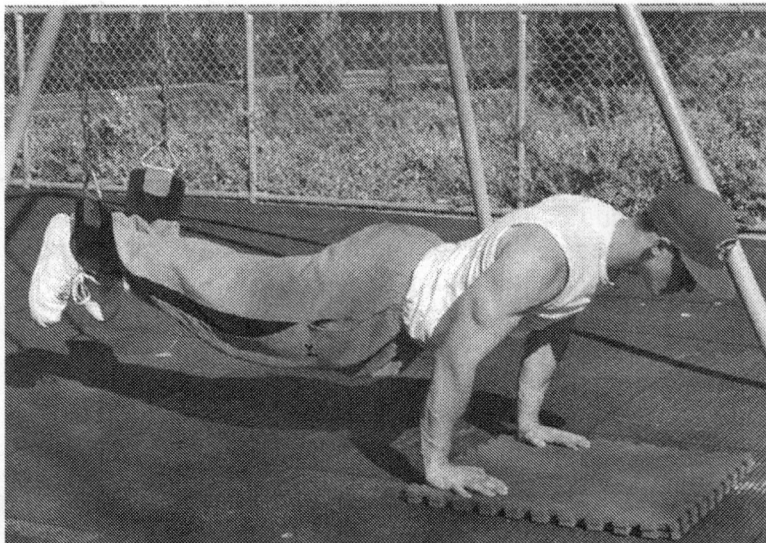

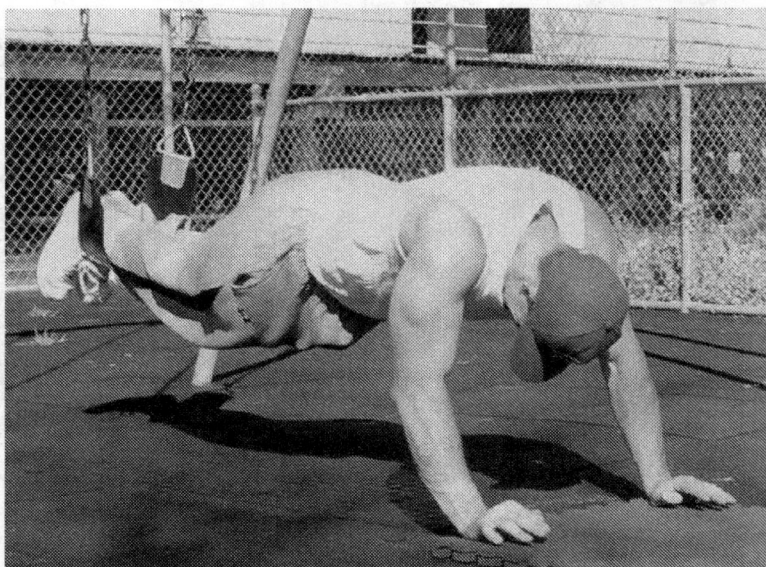

Always keep safety in mind!

Chest and Arms

As you pull the swing forward, try not to allow your lower back t drop lower than the height of the swing.

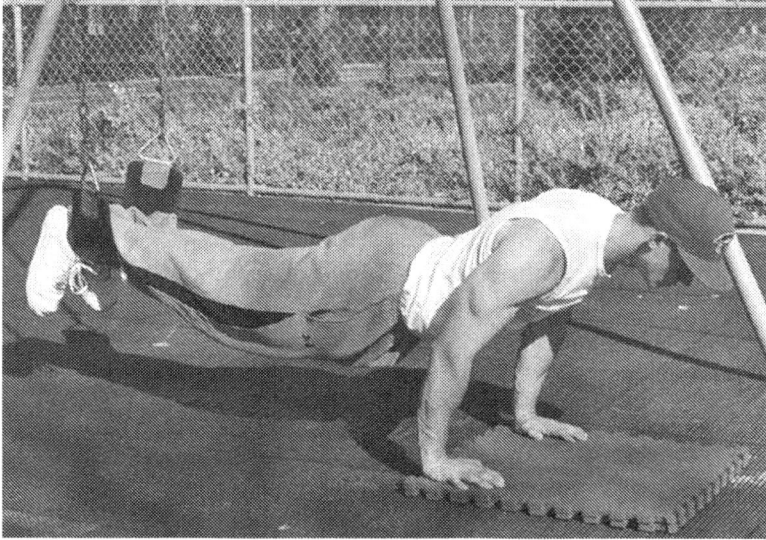

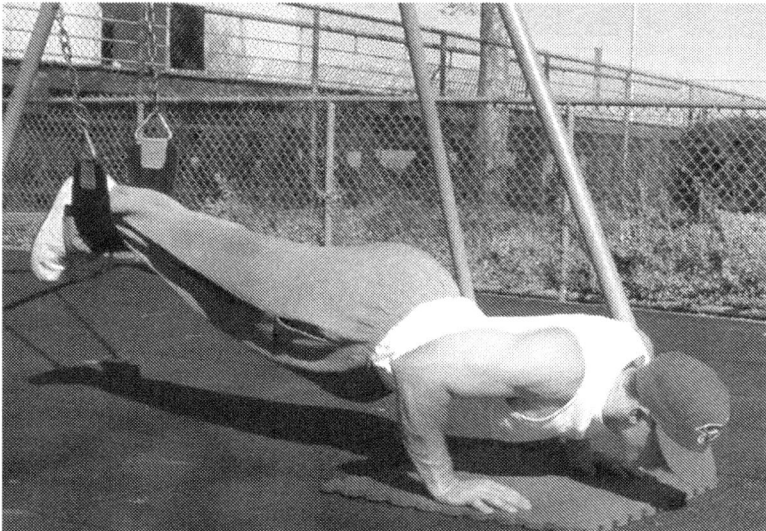

Explosive Push Ups

Start with your back facing the swing. Place your hands on the ground. Next, place your shins on the swing. You should be in a push up / plank position with your shins on the swing. Once positioned, lower your chest and chin toward the ground and then in an explosive motion, push your body up into the air. If performed correctly, your hands will leave the ground for the brief moment, because you have jumped. Make sure you bend your elbows immediately upon contact with the ground. Keep your core muscles tight and do not allow your lower back to hang down. Repeat for the desired number of repetitions. You should feel this in your chest, triceps, and core muscles.

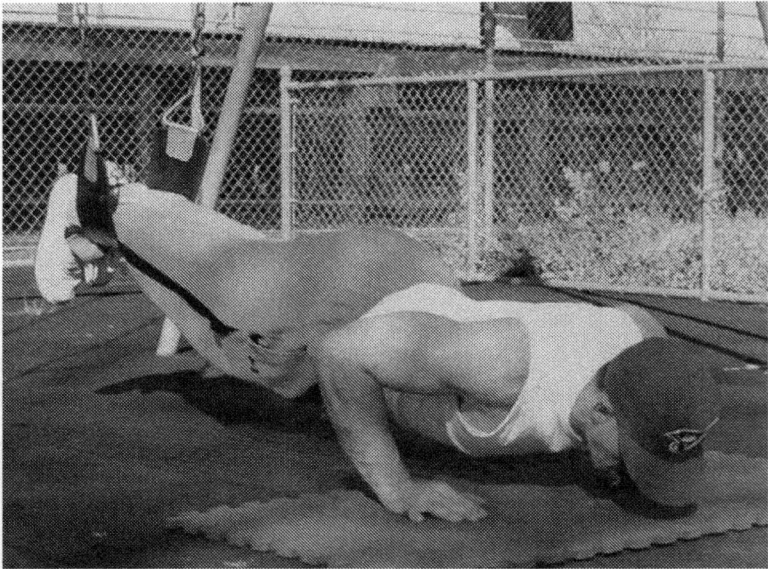

Chest and Arms

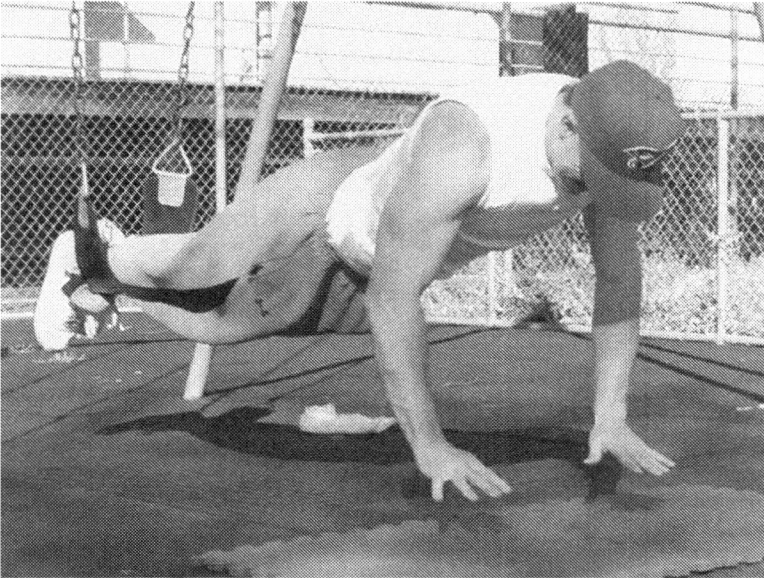

Make sure you bend your elbows immediately upon landing from the explosive pushup.

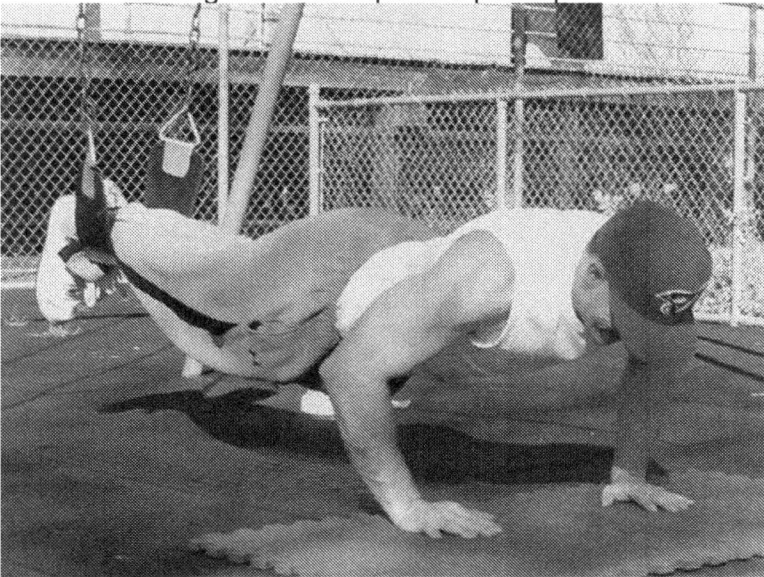

Triceps Extension (Swing)

Grasp the swing with both hands and position your forearms on the swing. Keeping your fingers wrapped around the bottom of the swing, raise the swing to chest height. Lean forward and allow the swing to help with balance. Lower your forearms to the swing for the starting position. Walk your feet backwards so that you are at a 45 degree angle. Next, lift your elbows up and then lower them back to the swing. You should feel this in your triceps. For a more intense triceps extension, walk your feet back so that your body more closely simulates a push up position.

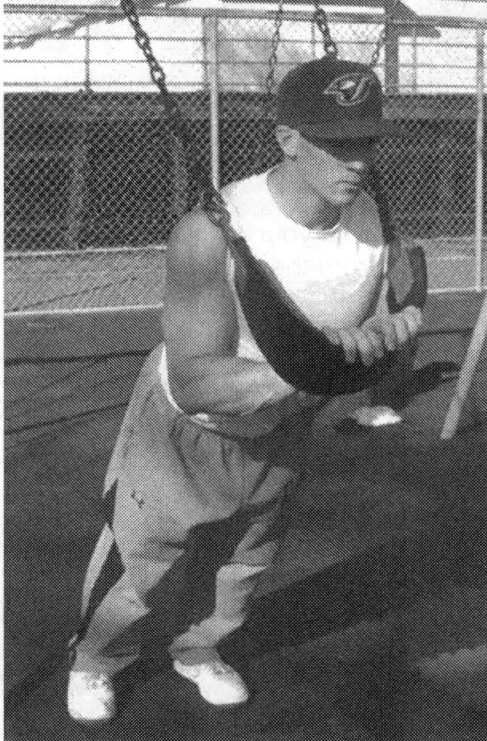

Always keep safety in mind!

Chest and Arms

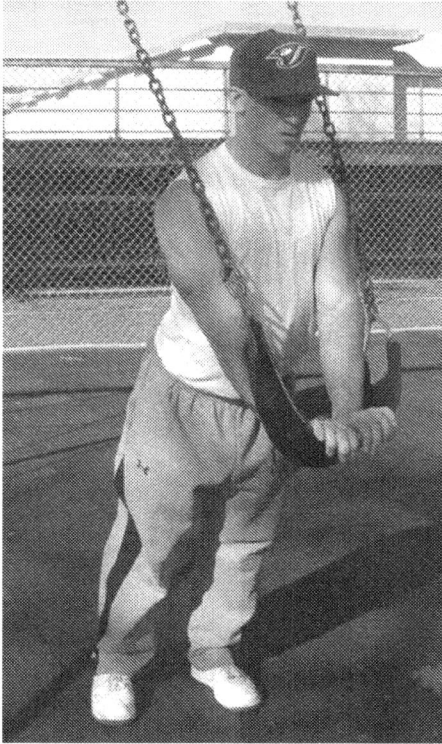

Swing Set Workouts

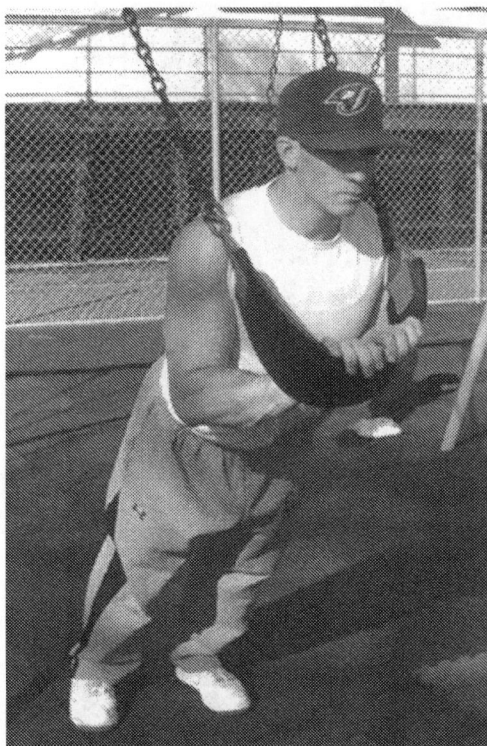

Always keep safety in mind!

Chest and Arms

Biceps Curl - Narrow

Grasp the bottom of the swing with both hands and wrap your fingers over the swing. The small fingers on each hand should be near each other to form a narrow grip. Keep your fingers wrapped around the bottom of the swing securely. Lean backwards so that your arms start nearly straight and walk your feet forward so that you are standing at a 45 degree angle. Make sure your feet will not slide. Next, using your biceps pull your chest in towards the swing. Keep your body straight and elbows near your ribs throughout this exercise. Keep your shoulders still while pulling so that you are performing a bicep curl, not a pull up. Open your arms and repeat the curl for the desired number of repetitions. You should feel this in your biceps.

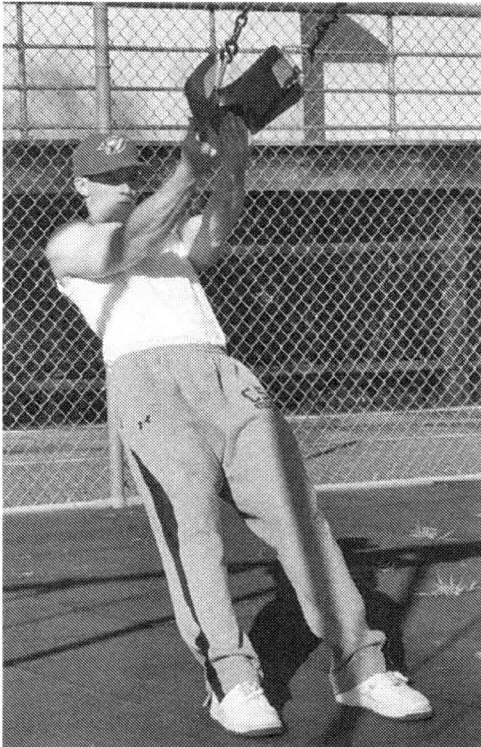

Swing Set Workouts

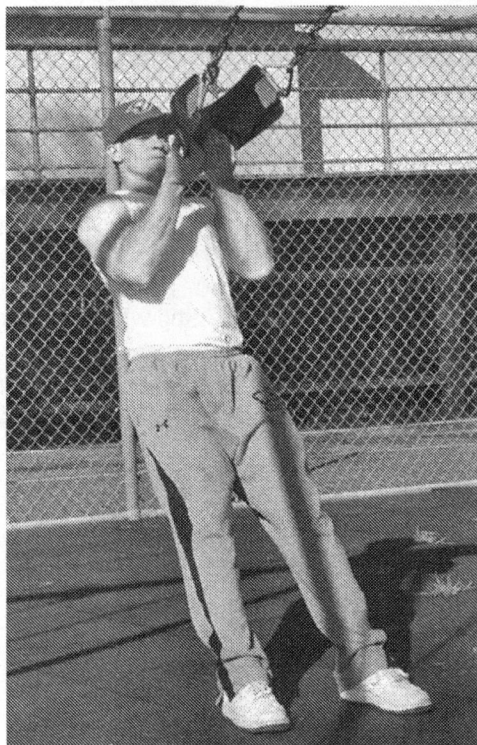

Always keep safety in mind!

Chest and Arms

Biceps Curl - Wide

Grasp the outer edges of the swing with both hands to
form a wide grip and wrap your fingers over the swing.
Keep your fingers wrapped around the swing securely.
Lean backwards so that your arms start nearly straight
and walk your feet forward so that you are standing at
a 45 degree angle. Make sure your feet will not slide.
Next, using your biceps pull your chest in towards the
swing. Keep your shoulders still while pulling so that
you are performing a bicep curl, not a pull up. Keep
your body straight throughout this exercise. Straighten
your arms and repeat the curl for the desired number
of repetition. You should feel this in your biceps.

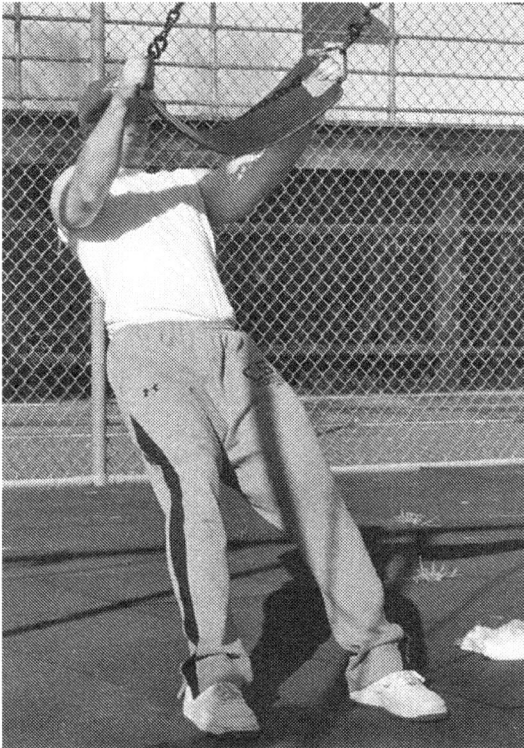

Swing Set Workouts

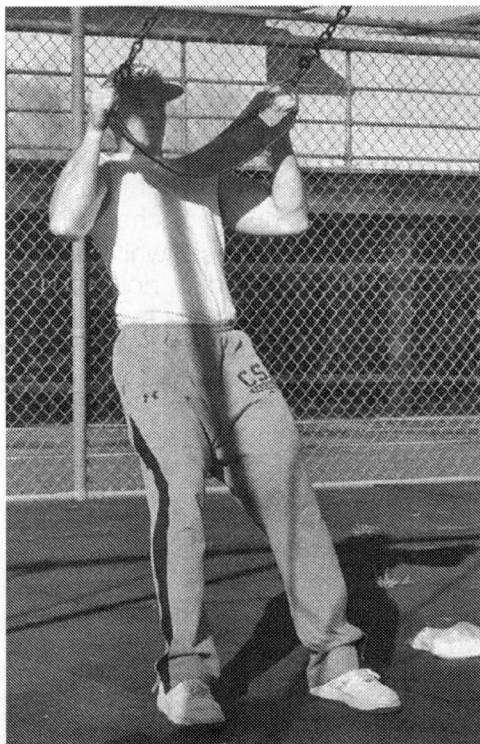

Always keep safety in mind!

Back and Biceps

This is an advanced workout. It is for people who train each body area one time per week using split routines. Your core muscles will be also become involved with some of the exercises included in this workout.

Three sets per exercise are recommended and 10-15 repetitions per set are appropriate for this type of workout. Perform no more than four sets per exercise.

Swing Set Workouts

Always keep safety in mind!

Back and Biceps

Straight Arm Lat Pull Down

Grasp the swing with both hands and position palms near the outer edge of swing. Keeping your fingers wrapped around the swing, raise the swing forward and up so that your arms are up by your ears. Your body will remain straight throughout this exercise. Lean forward and allow the swing to help with balance. Walk your feet backwards so that you are at an angle. Next, lower the swing forward and down so that the swing is below your ribs. Bring the swing back above your head and lower the swing again. You should feel this in your back, chest, and core muscles. It is similar to a straight arm dumbbell pullover or a kip motion.

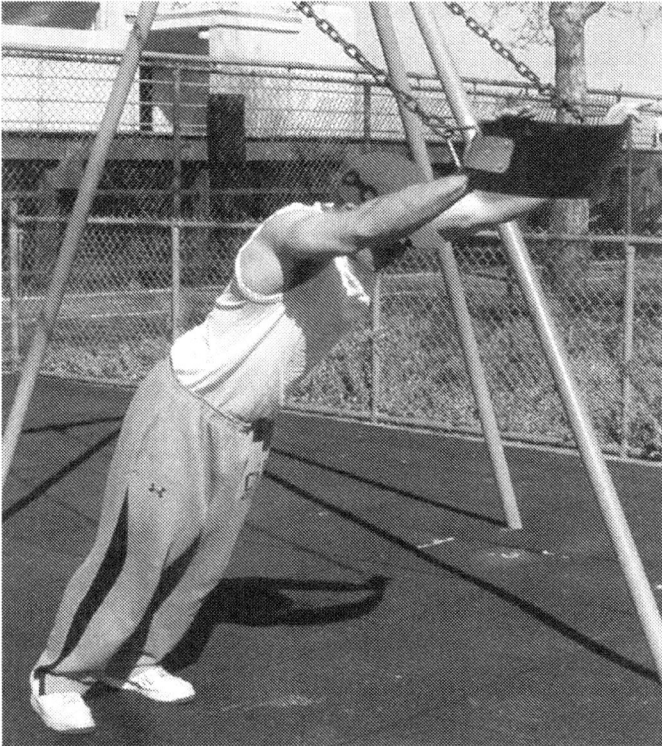

Swing Set Workouts

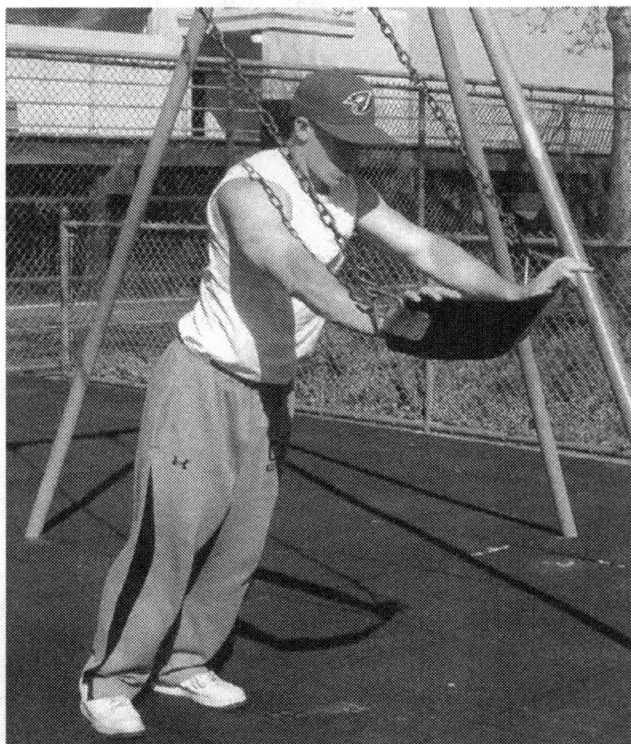

Always keep safety in mind!

Back and Biceps

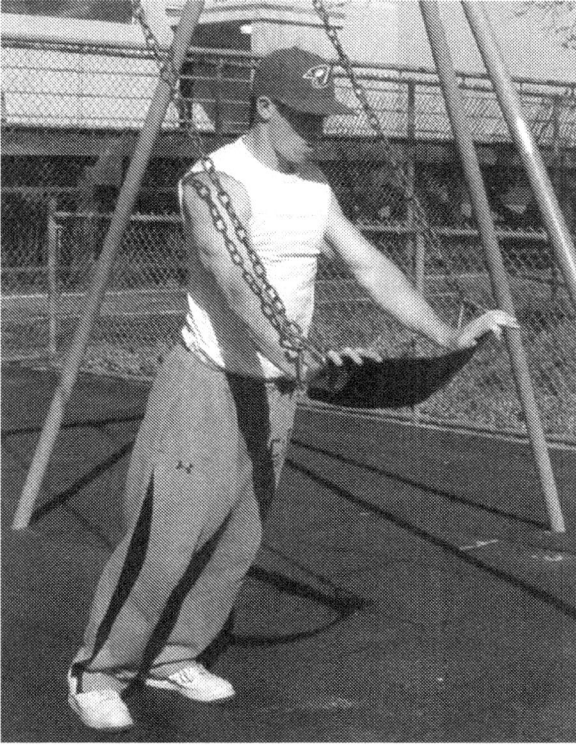

Modified Pull Up – Low

Grasp the outer portion of the swing with both hands and wrap fingers over the swing. Keeping your fingers wrapped around the bottom of the swing, lean backwards and walk your feet forward so that you are at a low position. Make sure your feet will not slide. Next, pull your chest in toward the swing. Keep your body straight throughout this exercise. You should feel this in your back and biceps.

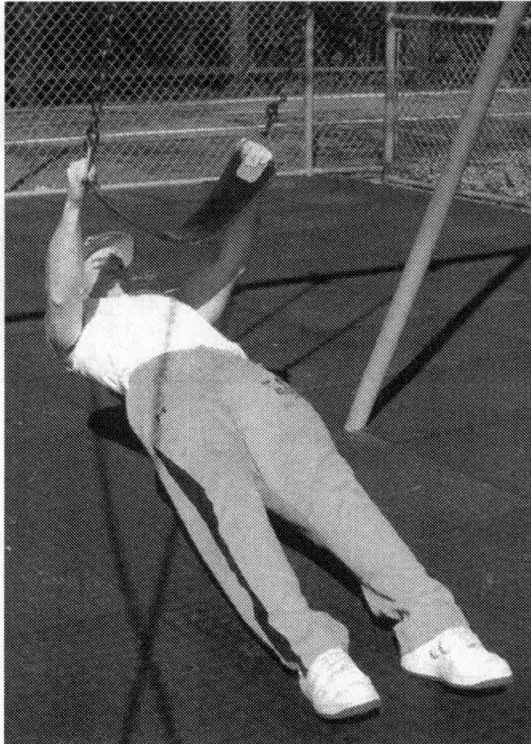

Always keep safety in mind!

Back and Biceps

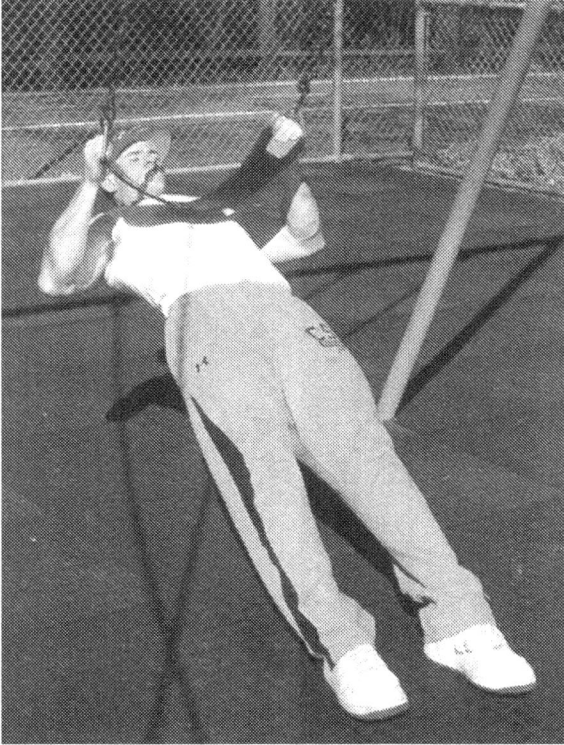

Modified Pull Up – High

Grasp the outer portion of the swing with both hands and wrap fingers over the swing. Keeping your fingers wrapped around the bottom of the swing, lean backward and move your feet forward so that you are at a slight angle. Make sure your feet will not slide. Next, pull your chest in towards the swing. Keep your body straight throughout this exercise. You should feel this in your back and biceps.

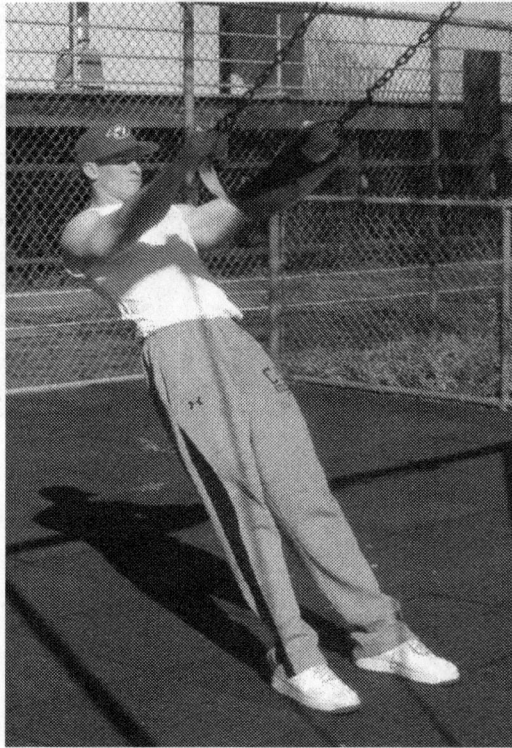

Always keep safety in mind!

Back and Biceps

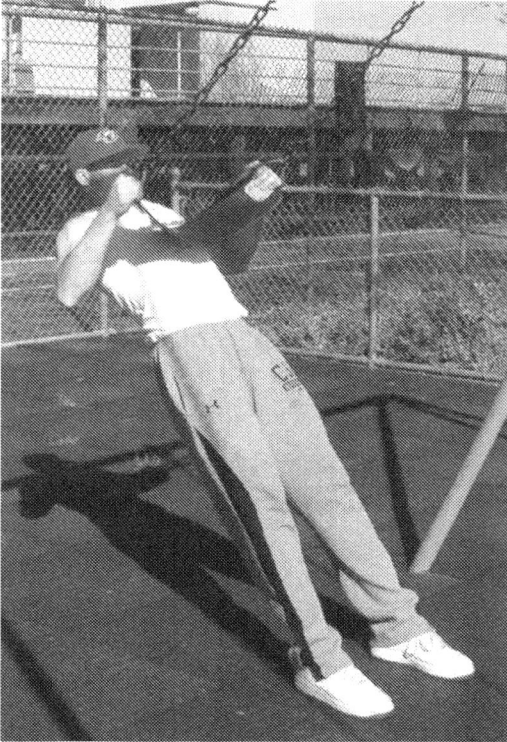

Swing Set Workouts

Biceps Curl - Narrow

Grasp the bottom of the swing with both hands and wrap your fingers over the swing. The small fingers on each hand should be near each other to form a narrow grip. Keep your fingers wrapped around the bottom of the swing securely. Lean backwards so that your arms start nearly straight and walk your feet forward so that you are standing at a 45 degree angle. Make sure your feet will not slide. Next, using your biceps pull your chest in towards the swing. Keep your body straight and elbows near your ribs throughout this exercise. Keep your shoulders still while pulling so that you are performing a bicep curl, not a pull up. Open your arms and repeat the curl for the desired number of repetitions. You should feel this in your biceps.

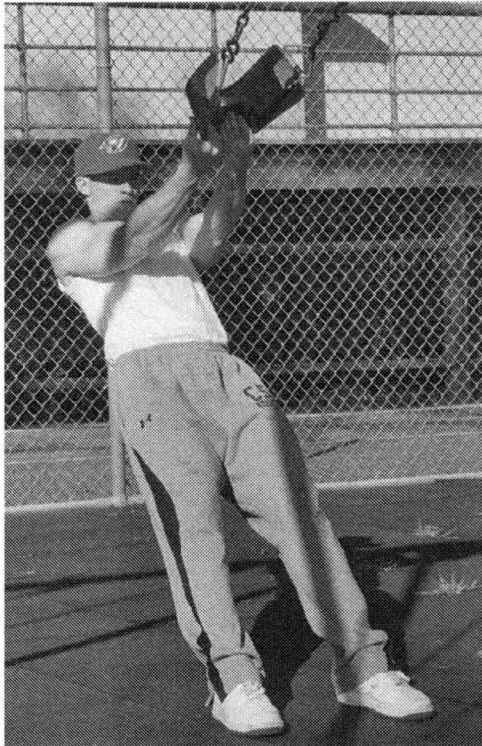

Always keep safety in mind!

Back and Biceps

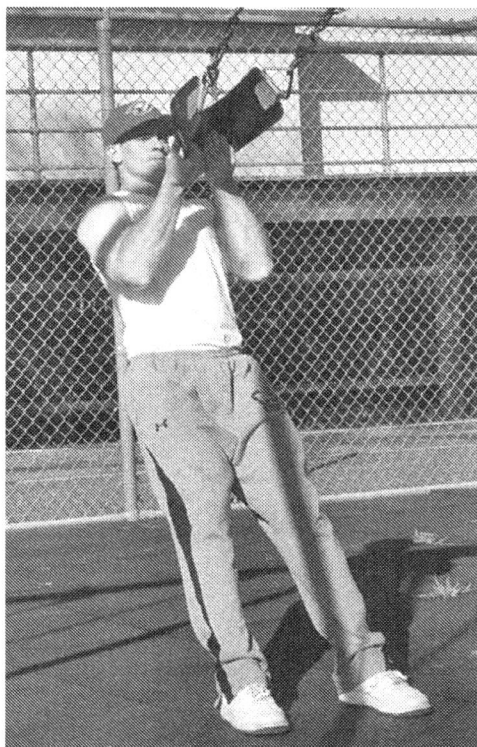

Biceps Curl - Wide
Grasp the outer edges of the swing with both hands to form a wide grip and wrap your fingers over the swing. Keep your fingers wrapped around the swing securely. Lean backwards so that your arms start nearly straight and walk your feet forward so that you are standing at a 45 degree angle. Make sure your feet will not slide. Next, using your biceps pull your chest in towards the swing. Keep your shoulders still while pulling so that you are performing a bicep curl, not a pull up. Keep your body straight throughout this exercise. Straighten your arms and repeat the curl for the desired number of repetition. You should feel this in your biceps.

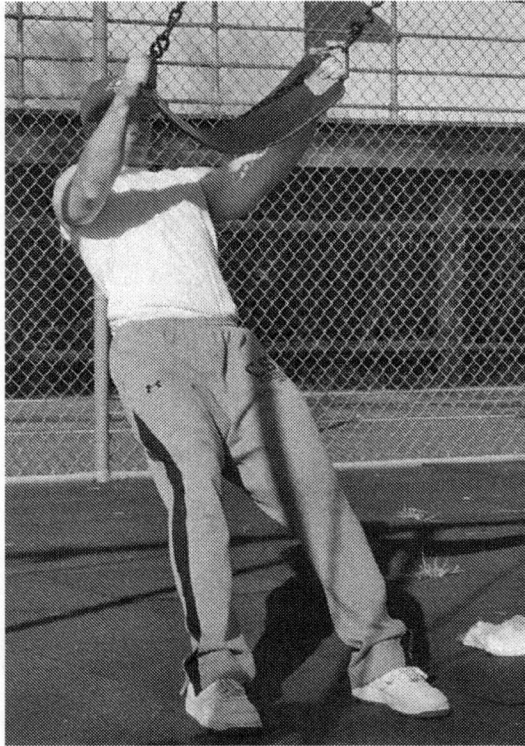

Always keep safety in mind!

Back and Biceps

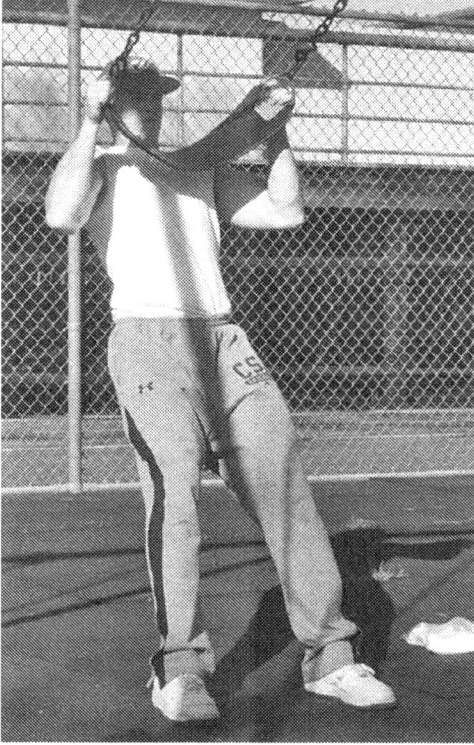

Swing Set Workouts

Swing Rocks / Pulls in Push Up Position

Start with your back facing the swing. Place your hands on the ground. Next, place your shins in the swing. You should be in a push up / plank position with your shins on the swing. Keep your hands in place in place on the ground and your arms straight throughout the exercise. Rock the swing forward and back. You will be pulling forward using your back / latissimus muscles and pushing backward using your shoulders. You should feel this in your chest, triceps, and shoulders, and core muscles. Repeat the swing rocks for the desired number of repetitions.

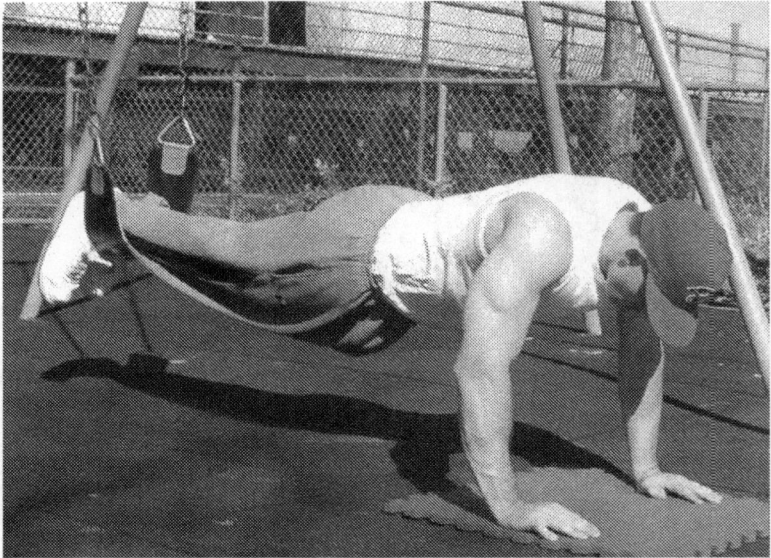

Always keep safety in mind!

Back and Biceps

As you pull the swing forward, try not to allow your lower back t drop lower than the height of the swing.

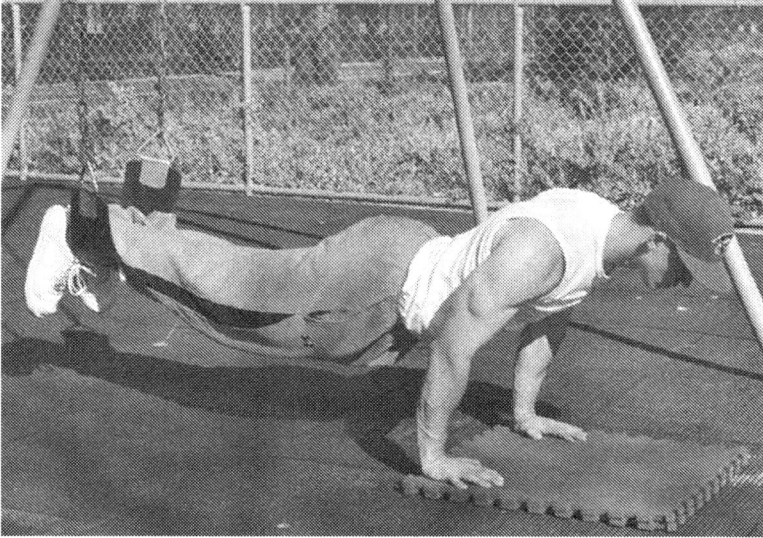

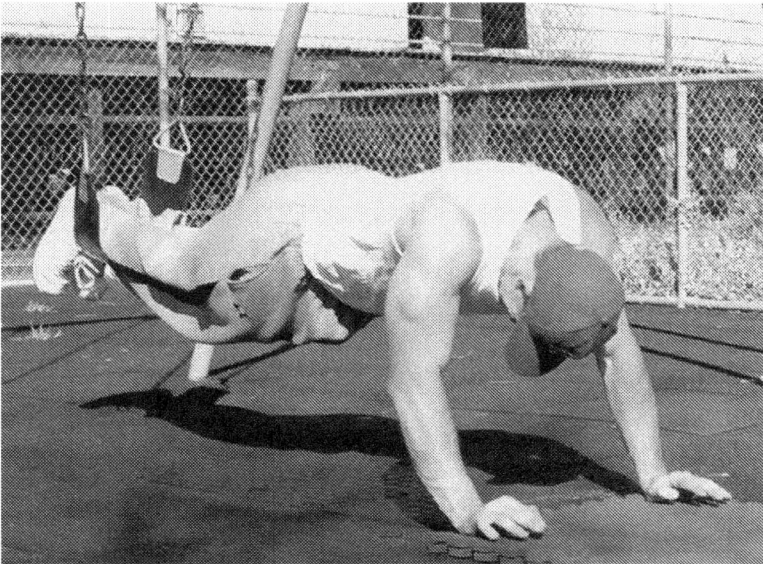

Chest and Triceps

This is an advanced workout. It is for people who train each body area one time per week using split routines. Your core muscles will be also become involved with some of the exercises included in this workout.

Three sets per exercise are recommended and 10-15 repetitions per set are appropriate for this type of workout. Perform no more than four sets per exercise.

Swing Set Workouts

Always keep safety in mind!

Chest and Triceps

Swing Walks - Forward and Back

Start with your back facing the swing. Place your hands on the ground. Next, place your shins on the swing. You should be in a push up / plank position with your shins on the swing. Keep your arms straight throughout the exercise. Walk your hands forward as far as possible and then walk backward as far as possible. You will be pulling forward using your back / latissimus muscles and pushing backward using your shoulders. It will be slightly more difficult than the swing rocks because you will be pulling and pushing with one the muscles on one side at a time. You will also be supporting your body with one side at a time as you shift your weight from one hand to the other. You should feel this in your chest, shoulders, back, triceps, and core muscles. Repeat the swing walks for the desired number of repetitions.

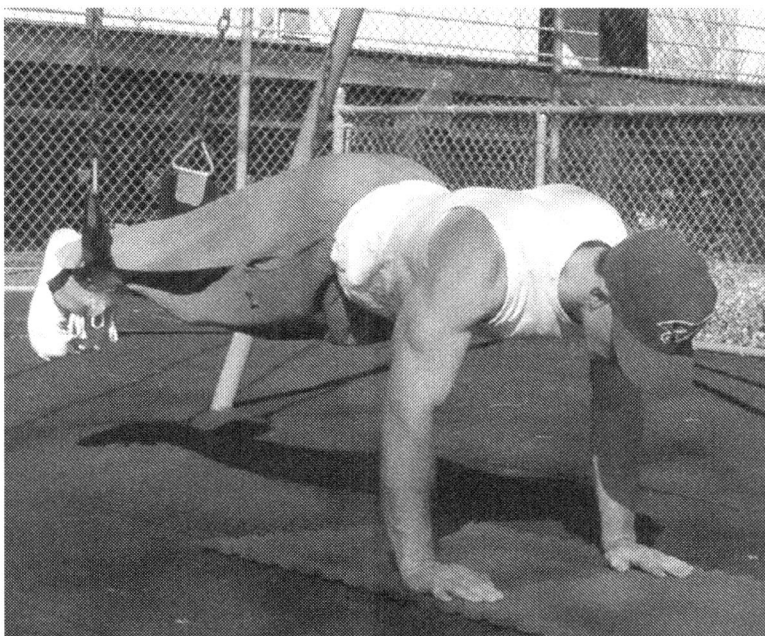

Swing Set Workouts

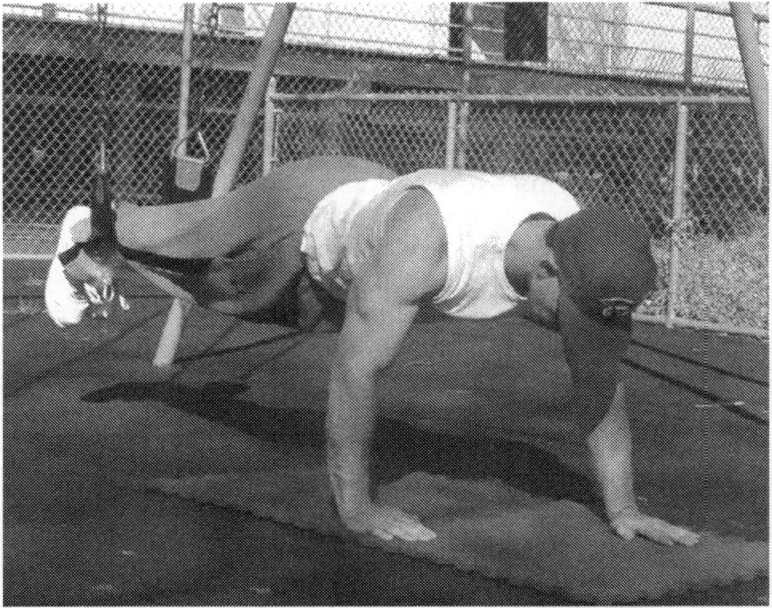

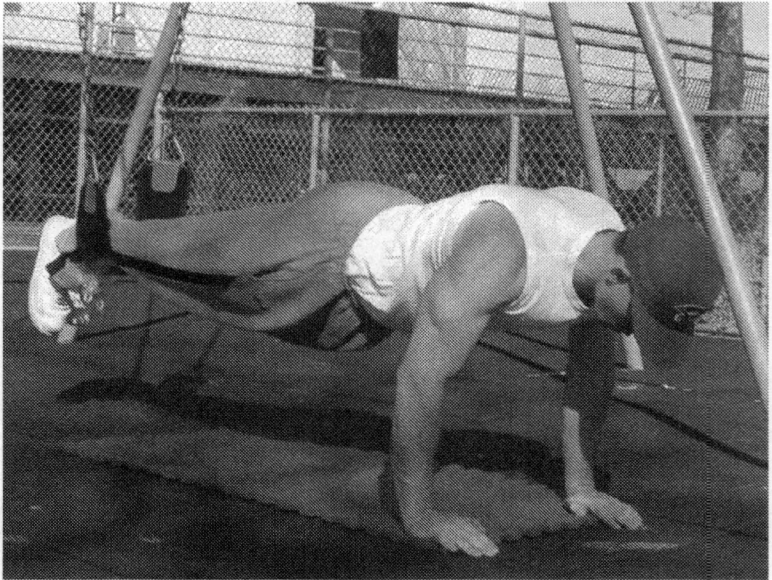

Always keep safety in mind!

Chest and Triceps

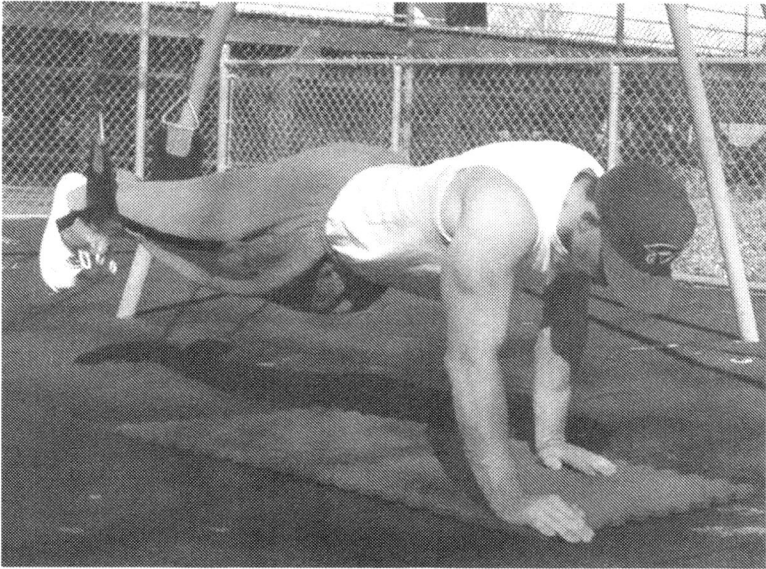

Swing Push Ups – Shins on Swing
Start with your back facing the swing. Place your hands on the ground. Next, place your shins on the swing. You should be in a push up position with your shins on the swing. Once positioned, lower your chest and chin near the ground and then push back up. Keep your core muscles tight and do not allow your lower back to hang down. Repeat for the desired number of repetitions. You should feel this in your chest, triceps, and core muscles.

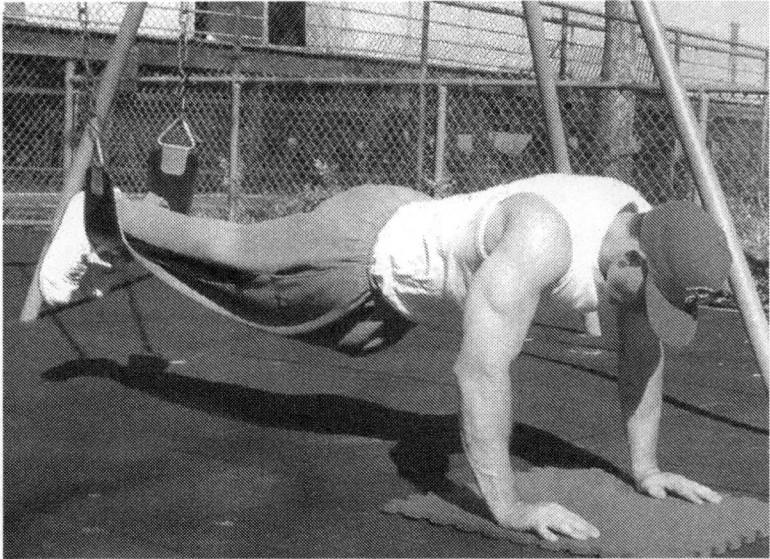

Chest and Triceps

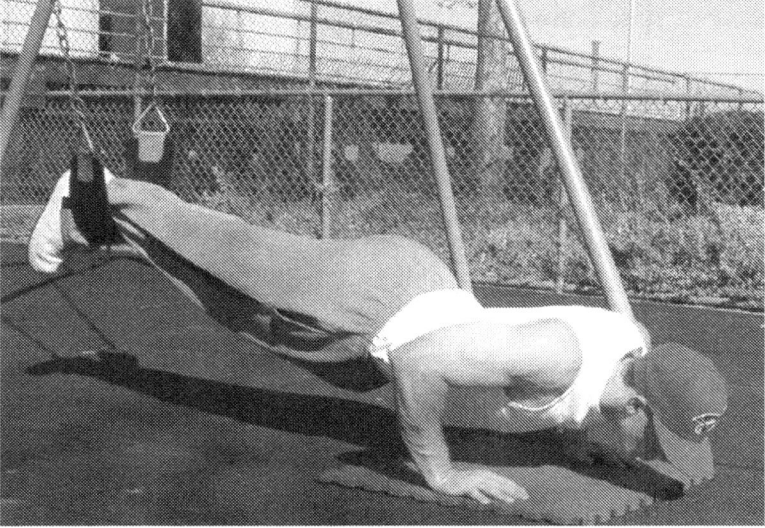

Swing Set Workouts

Explosive Push Ups

Start with your back facing the swing. Place your hands on the ground. Next, place your shins on the swing. You should be in a push up / plank position with your shins on the swing. Once positioned, lower your chest and chin toward the ground and then in an explosive motion, push your body up into the air. If performed correctly, your hands will leave the ground for the brief moment, because you have jumped. Make sure you bend your elbows immediately upon contact with the ground. Keep your core muscles tight and do not allow your lower back to hang down. Repeat for the desired number of repetitions. You should feel this in your chest, triceps, and core muscles.

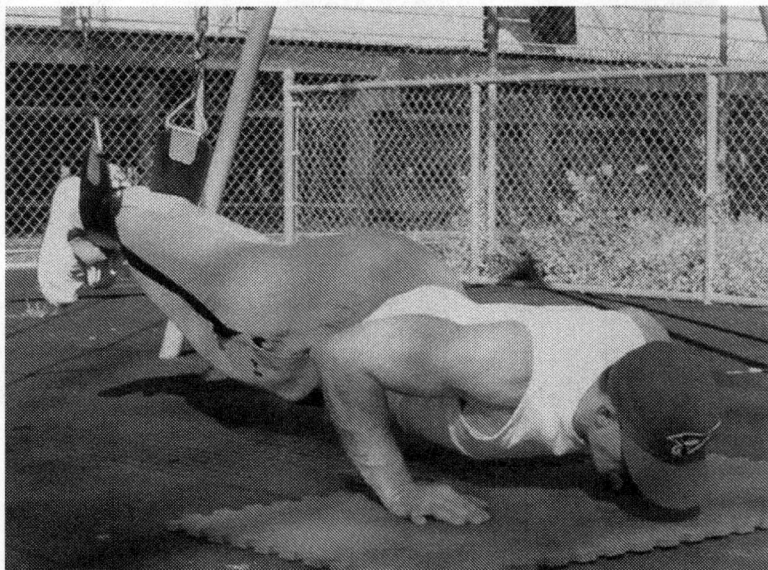

Always keep safety in mind!

Chest and Triceps

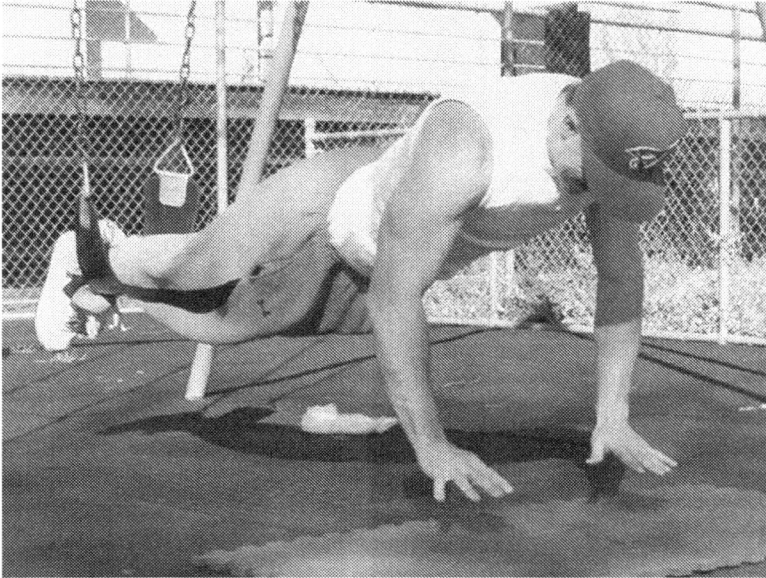

Make sure you bend your elbows immediately upon landing from the explosive pushup.

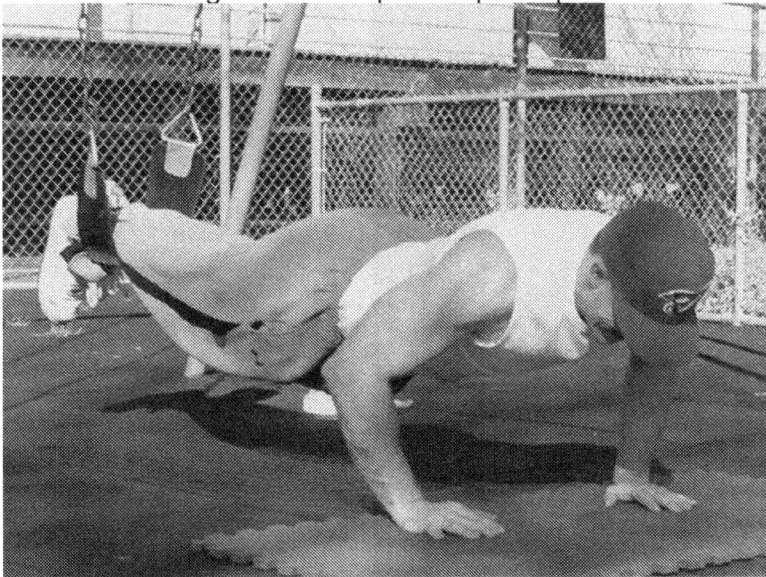

Swing Set Workouts

Swing Protraction / Shrugs (Ground)

Start with your back facing the swing. Place your hands on the ground. Next, place your shins on the swing. You should be in a push up / plank position with your shins on the swing. Keep your back straight and your core muscles tight. Once in position, pull in your chest and raise your upper back toward the sky.

The portion of your back between your shoulder blades will become rounded. Return top the flat back push up position and press up again. It is a chest and shoulder motion. Your arms remain straight. Repeat he protractions for the desired the desired number of repetitions. This exercise can be preformed with your forearms and palms on the ground. You should feel this in your chest, triceps, and core muscles.

This exercise can be performed on your forearms to change the angle and muscle demand. It is also a great alternative if your wrists are sore.

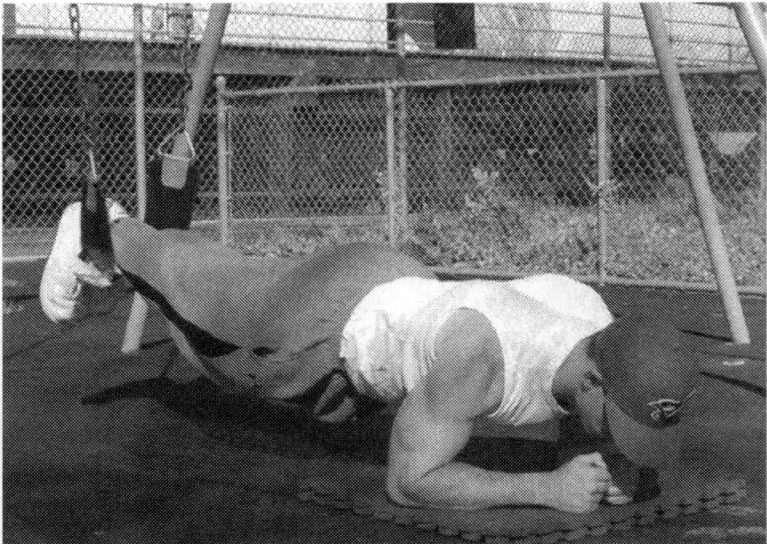

Always keep safety in mind!

Chest and Triceps

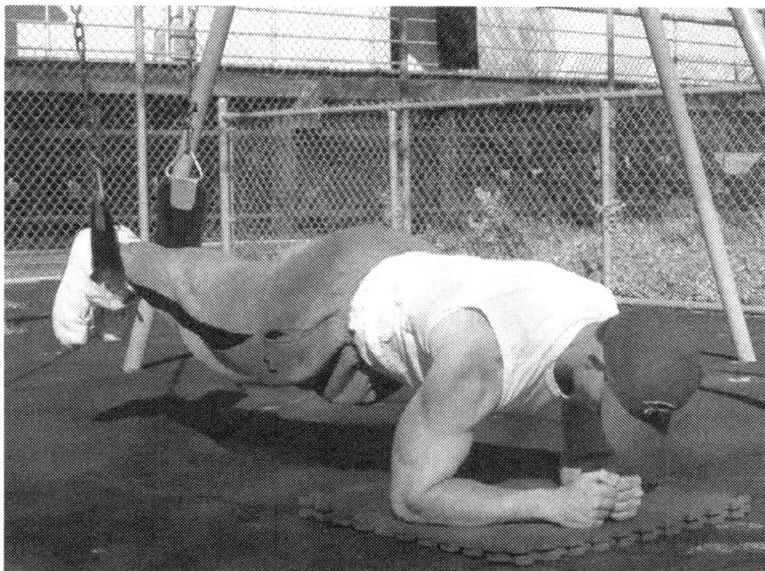

Advanced Triceps Extension (Ground)

Start with your back facing the swing. Place your hands on the ground. Next, place your shins on the swing. You should be in a push up position with your shins on the swing. Once in position, lower your elbows to the ground and lift them up again. Keep your elbows in line with your ribs. This is not a push up. You are lowering and lifting your elbows. Do not allow your elbows to hit or scrape the ground. If it is too difficult to lower and lift both elbows at the same time, lower and lift one elbow at a time, alternating sides. You should feel this in your triceps and core muscles.

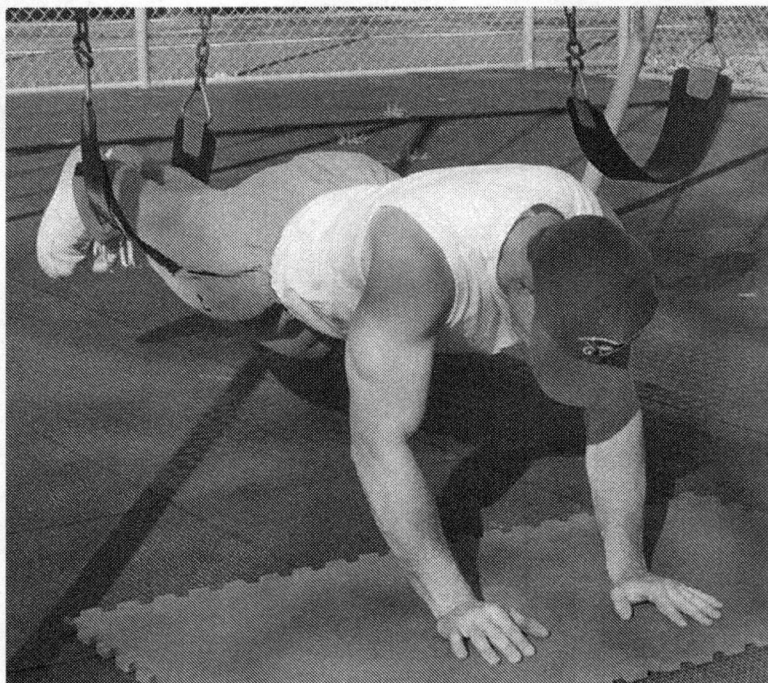

Always keep safety in mind!

Chest and Triceps

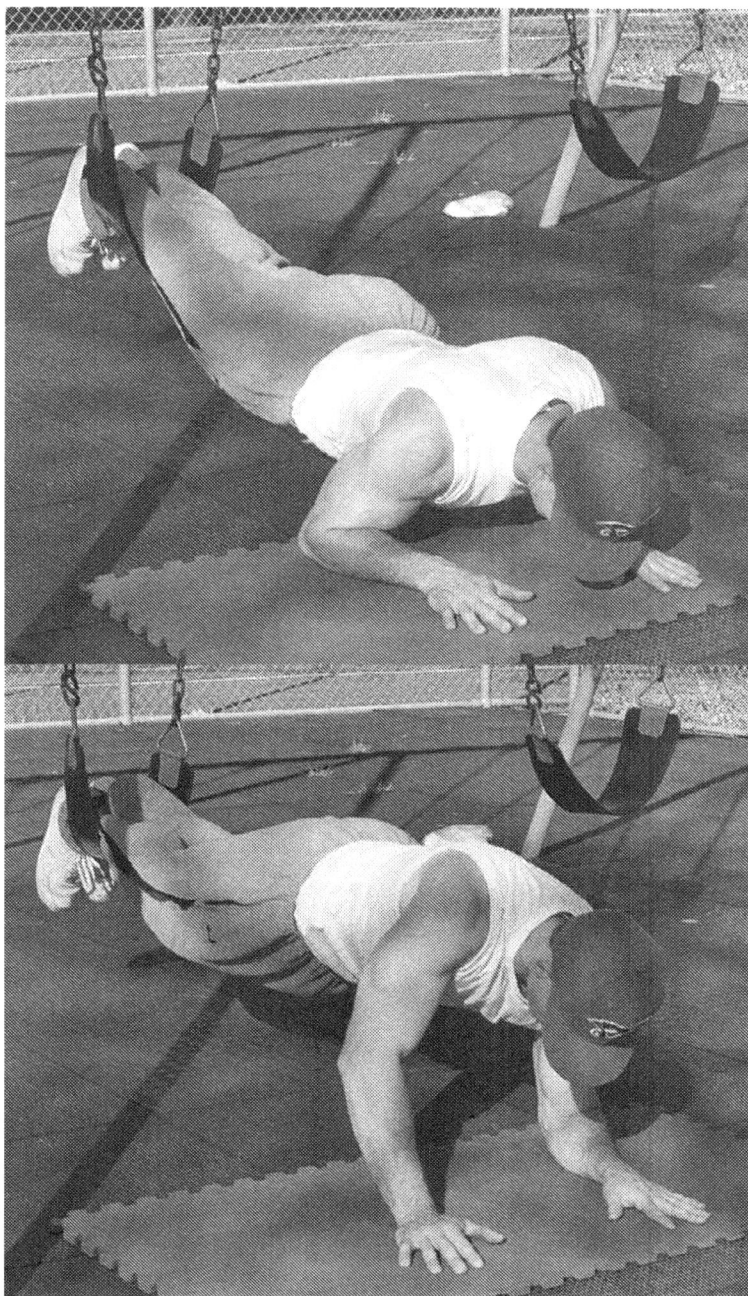

Triceps Extension (Swing)

Grasp the swing with both hands and position your forearms on the swing. Keeping your fingers wrapped around the bottom of the swing, raise the swing to chest height. Lean forward and allow the swing to help with balance. Lower your forearms to the swing for the starting position. Walk your feet backwards so that you are at a 45 degree angle. Next, lift your elbows up and then lower them back to the swing. You should feel this in your triceps. For a more intense triceps extension, walk your feet back so that your body more closely simulates a push up position.

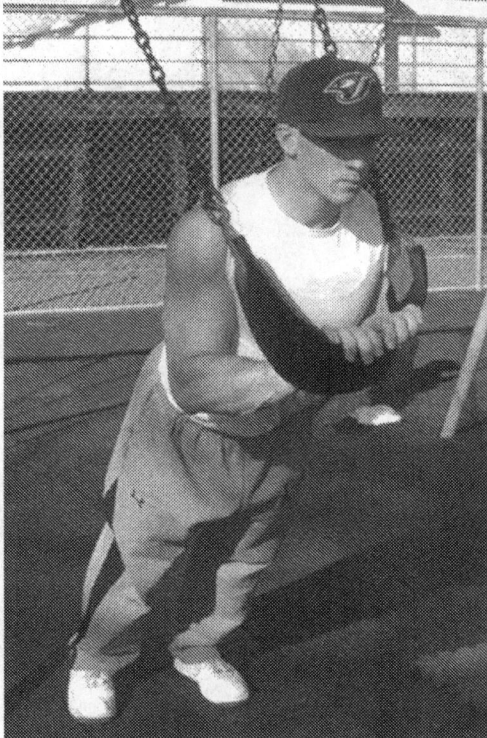

Always keep safety in mind!

Chest and Triceps

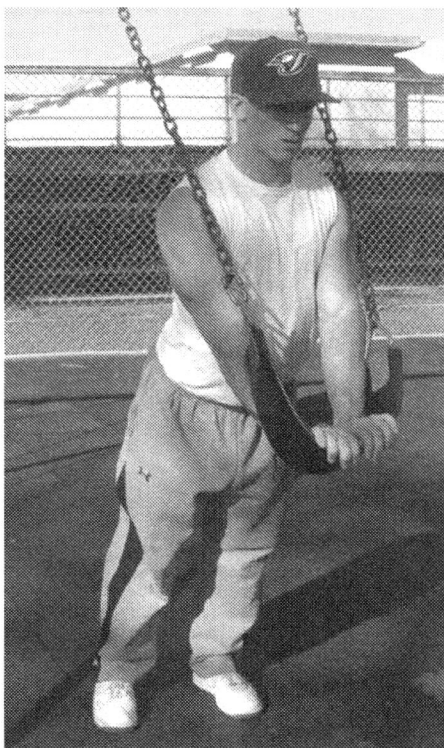

Swing Set Workouts

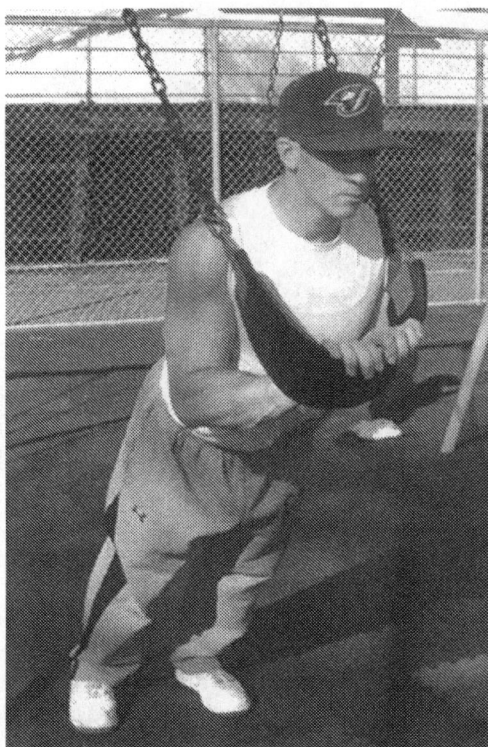

Always keep safety in mind!

Chest and Shoulders

This is an advanced workout. It is for people who train each body area one time per week using split routines. Your core muscles will be also become involved with some of the exercises included in this workout.

Three sets per exercise are recommended and 10-15 repetitions per set are appropriate for this type of workout. Perform no more than four sets per exercise.

Chest and Shoulders

Swing Rocks / Pulls in Push Up Position

Start with your back facing the swing. Place your hands on the ground. Next, place your shins in the swing. You should be in a push up / plank position with your shins on the swing. Keep your hands in place in place on the ground and your arms straight throughout the exercise. Rock the swing forward and back. You will be pulling forward using your back / latissimus muscles and pushing backward using your shoulders. You should feel this in your chest, triceps, and shoulders, and core muscles. Repeat the swing rocks for the desired number of repetitions.

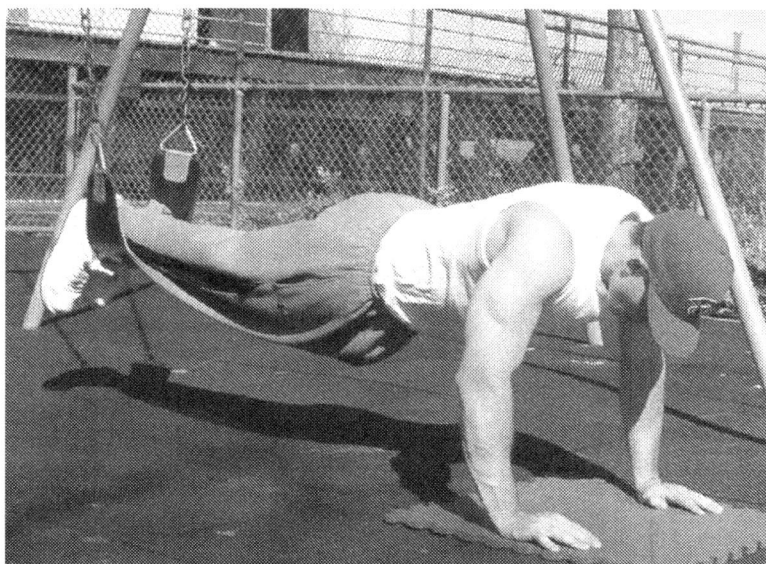

Swing Set Workouts

As you pull the swing forward, try not to allow your lower back t drop lower than the height of the swing.

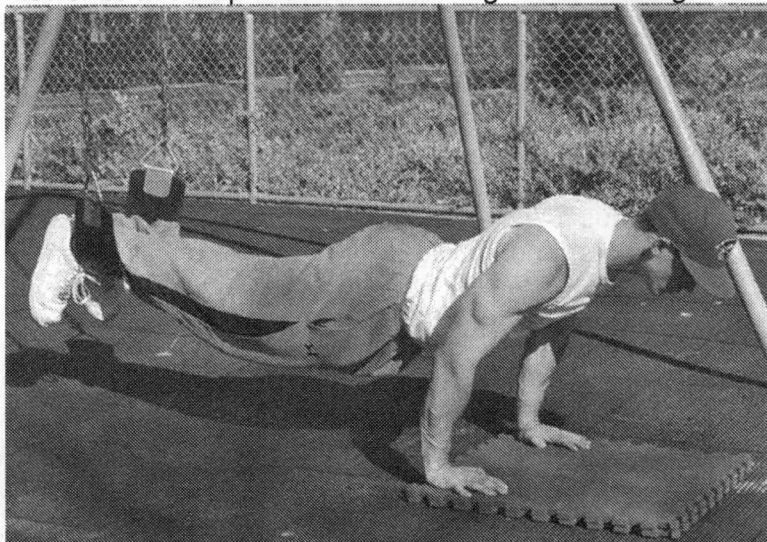

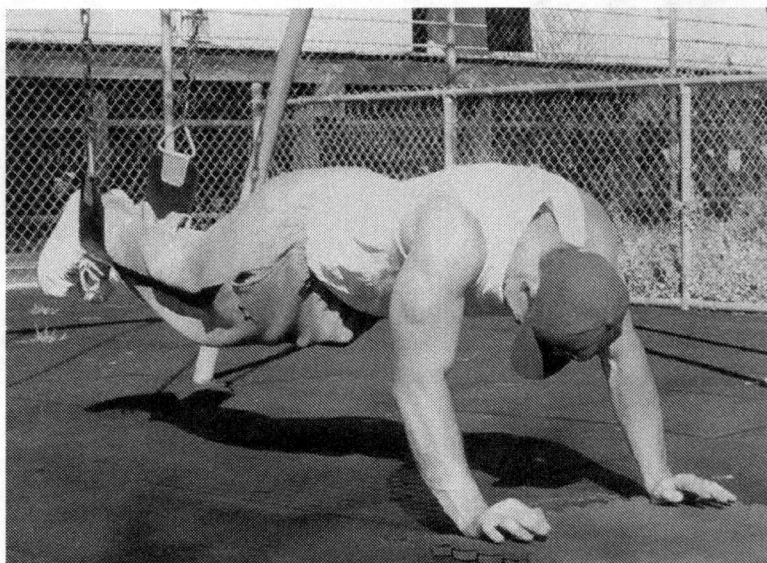

Always keep safety in mind!

Chest and Shoulders

Swing Rocks / Pulls with Push Up

Start with your back facing the swing. Place your hands on the ground. Next, place your shins on the swing. You should be in a push up / plank position with your shins on the swing. Keep your hands in place on the ground and your arms straight during the rock portion. Rock the swing forward and back two times. You will be pulling forward using your back / latissimus muscles and pushing backward using your shoulders. On the second forward rock of the swing, when your shoulders are beyond your hands, perform two push ups. Rock again and then perform another two push ups. You should feel this in your chest, triceps, shoulders, and core muscles. Repeat the swing rock with push ups for the desired number of repetitions.

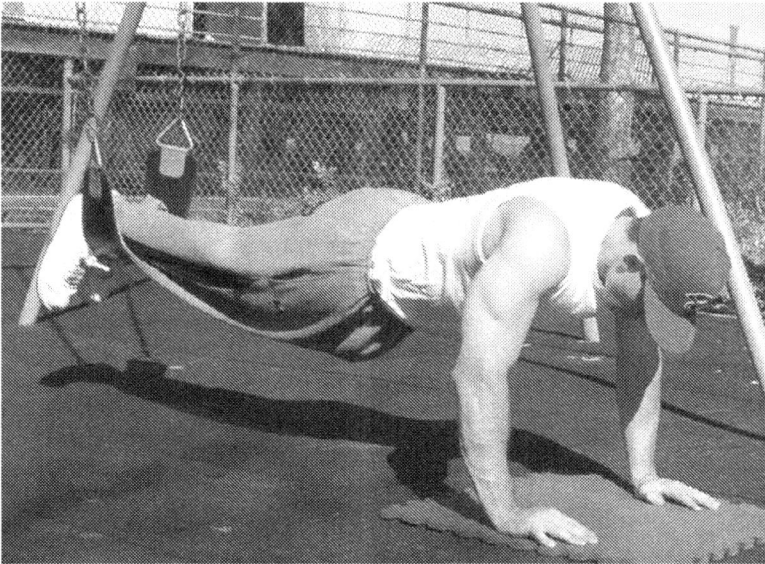

Swing Set Workouts

As you pull the swing forward, try not to allow your lower back t drop lower than the height of the swing.

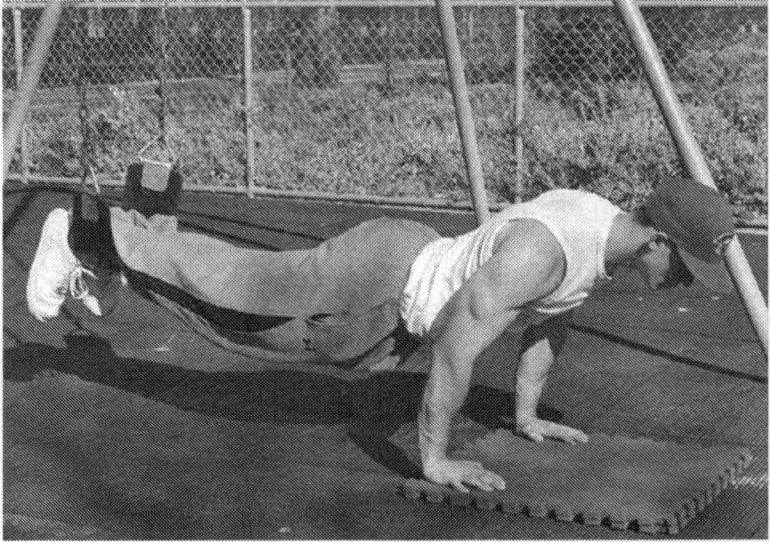

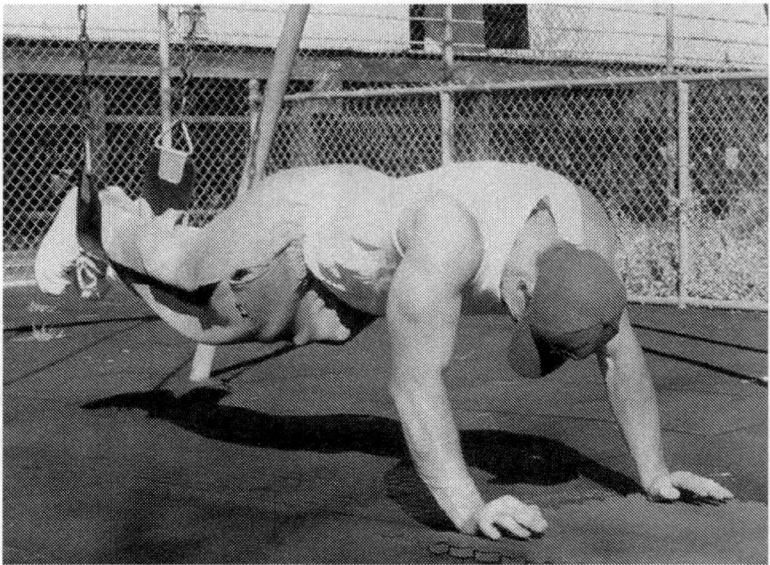

Always keep safety in mind!

Chest and Shoulders

As you pull the swing forward, try not to allow your lower back t drop lower than the height of the swing.

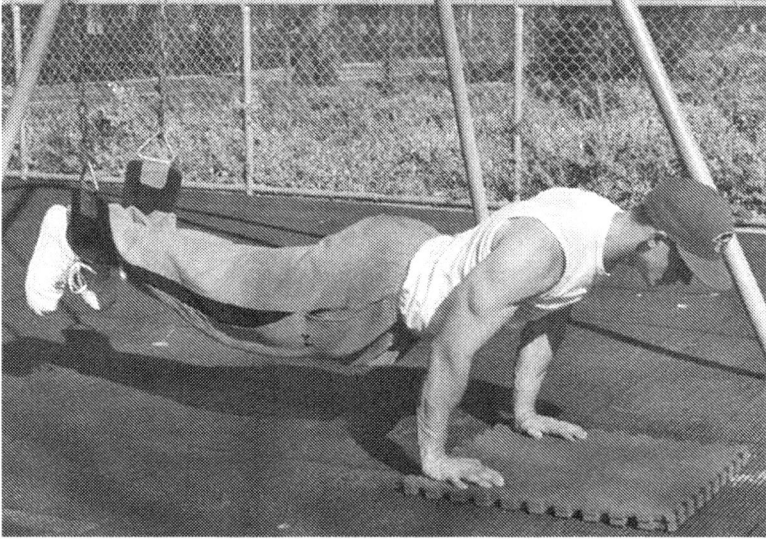

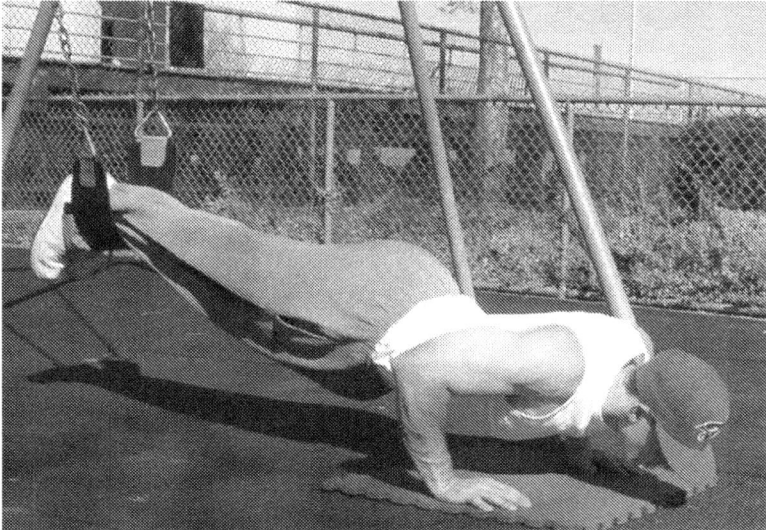

Swing Set Workouts

Explosive Push Ups

Start with your back facing the swing. Place your hands on the ground. Next, place your shins on the swing. You should be in a push up / plank position with your shins on the swing. Once positioned, lower your chest and chin toward the ground and then in an explosive motion, push your body up into the air. If performed correctly, your hands will leave the ground for the brief moment, because you have jumped. Make sure you bend your elbows immediately upon contact with the ground. Keep your core muscles tight and do not allow your lower back to hang down. Repeat for the desired number of repetitions. You should feel this in your chest, triceps, and core muscles.

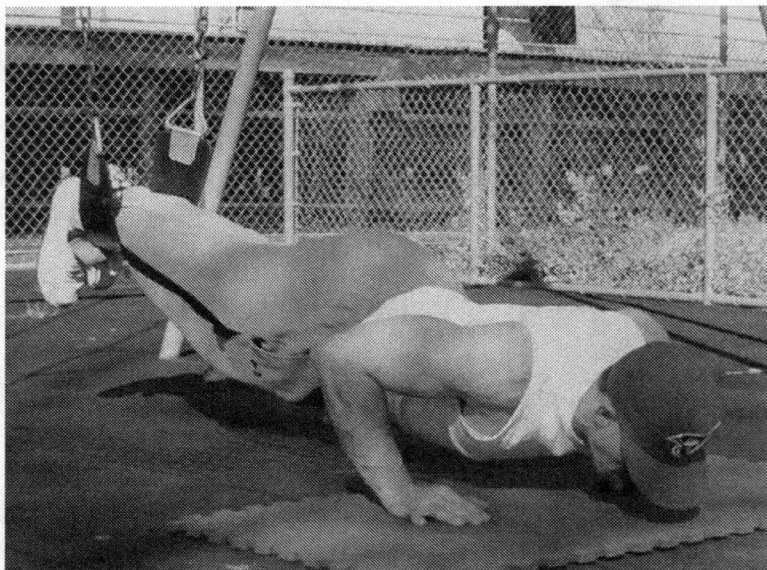

Always keep safety in mind!

Chest and Shoulders

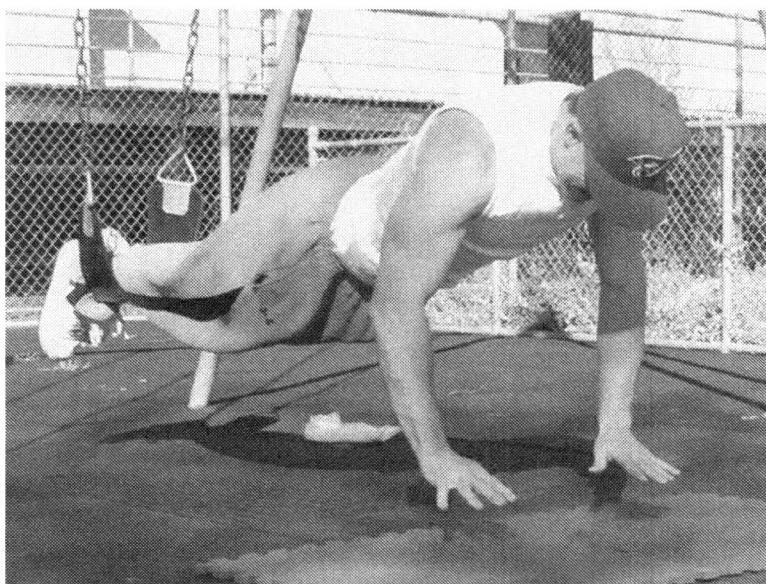

Make sure you bend your elbows immediately upon landing from the explosive pushup.

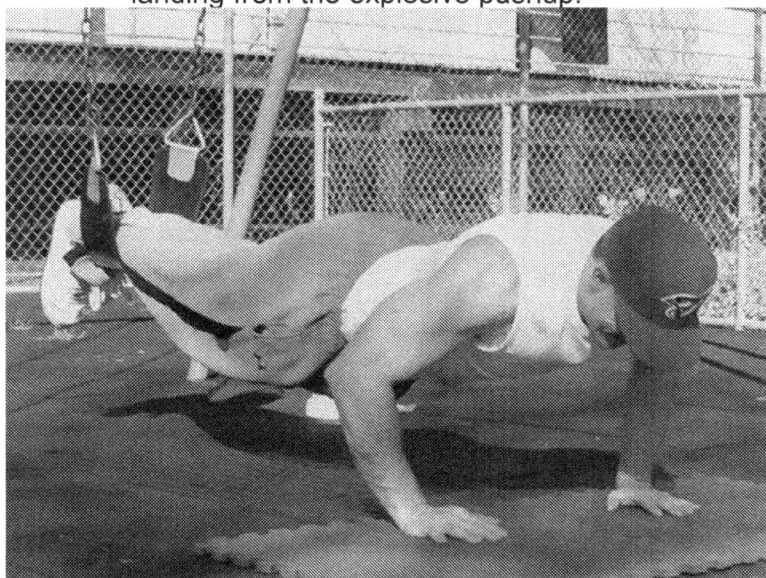

Swing Set Workouts

Pike / Virtual Handstand Push Up
Start with your back facing the swing. Place your hands on the ground. Next, place your shins on the swing. You should be in a push up / plank position with your shins on the swing. Next, pull your belly in so that you bend at the hips to form a full pike position, virtual handstand. Your hips will be directly above your head. Once in the virtual handstand, bend your elbows so that your head moves towards the ground. Do not allow your head to touch the ground! Your legs will remain straight. Your upper body will be in a virtual handstand during these push ups. Return to the virtual handstand and then to the straight push up / plank position. Repeat the handstand pushup for the desired number of repetitions. You should feel this in your shoulders and core muscles.

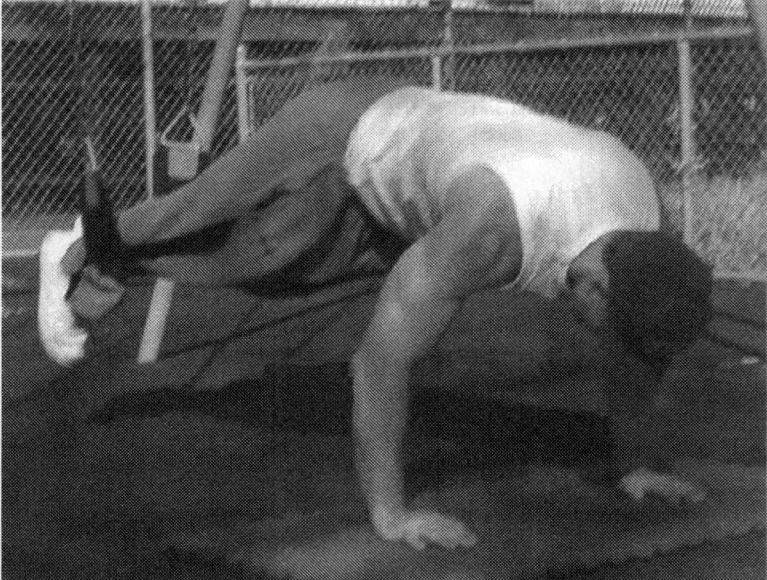

Always keep safety in mind!

Chest and Shoulders

Do not allow your head or face to contact the ground.
Only perform this exercise of you are strong enough to
support yourself upside down.

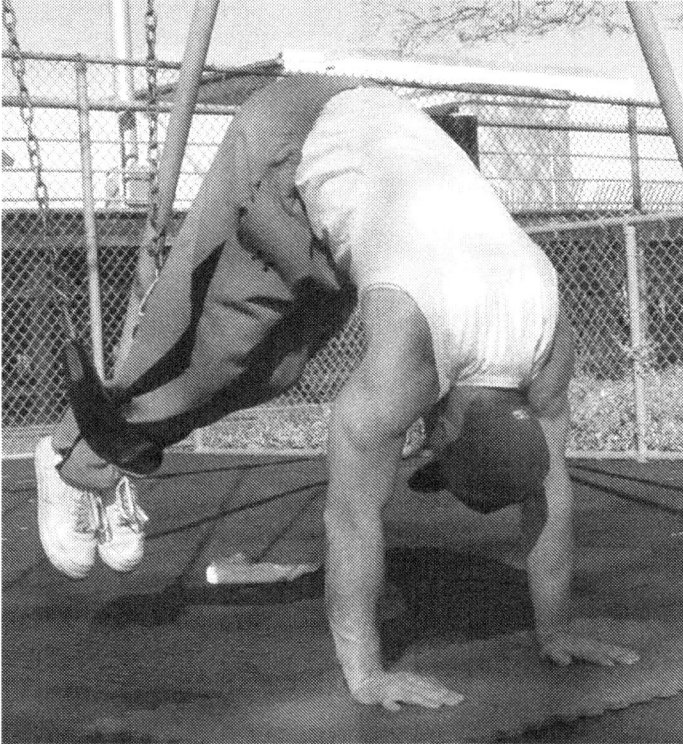

Swing Set Workouts

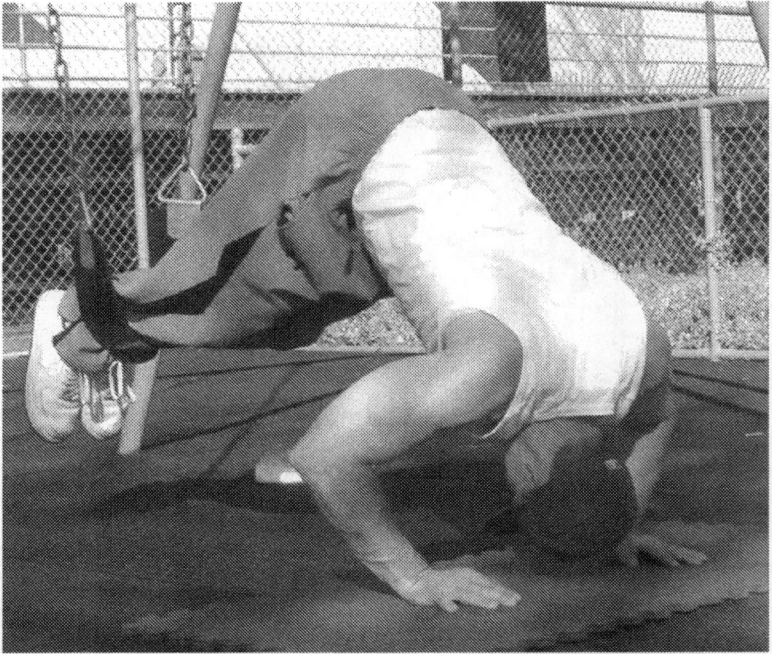

Always keep safety in mind!

Chest and Shoulders

Full Pike / Virtual Handstand with Shrug

Start with your back facing the swing. Place your hands on the ground. Next, place your shins on the swing. You should be in a push up / plank position with your shins on the swing. Next, pull your belly in so that you bend at the hips to form a full pike position, virtual handstand. Your hips will be directly above your head. Your legs and arms will remain straight. Your upper body will be in a virtual handstand. Once in the virtual handstand, shrug your shoulders so that your shoulders move toward your ears. Return to the straight push up / plank position and repeat the full pike and shrug for the desired number of repetitions. You should feel this in your core, chest, and shoulder muscles.

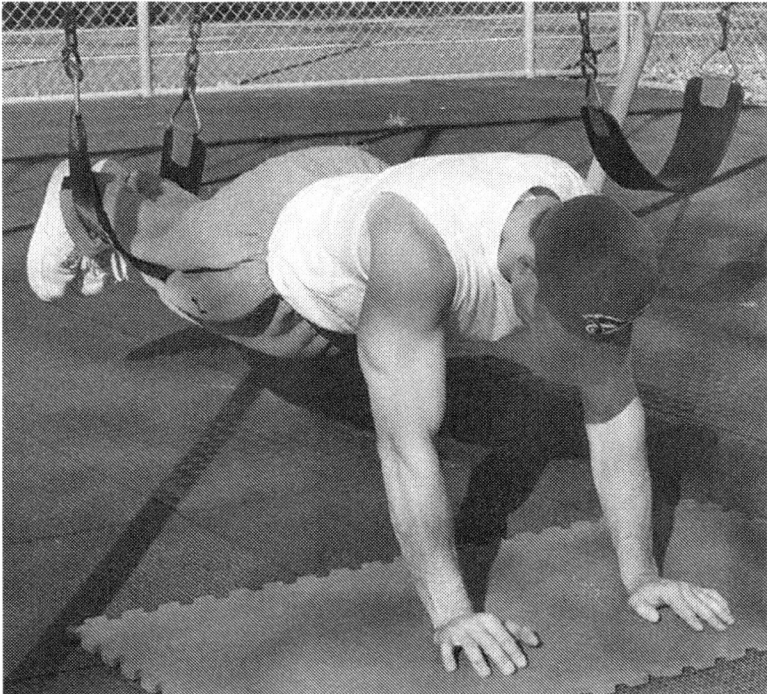

Swing Set Workouts

Only pull up to the full pike if you are strong enough to support your body weight upside down.

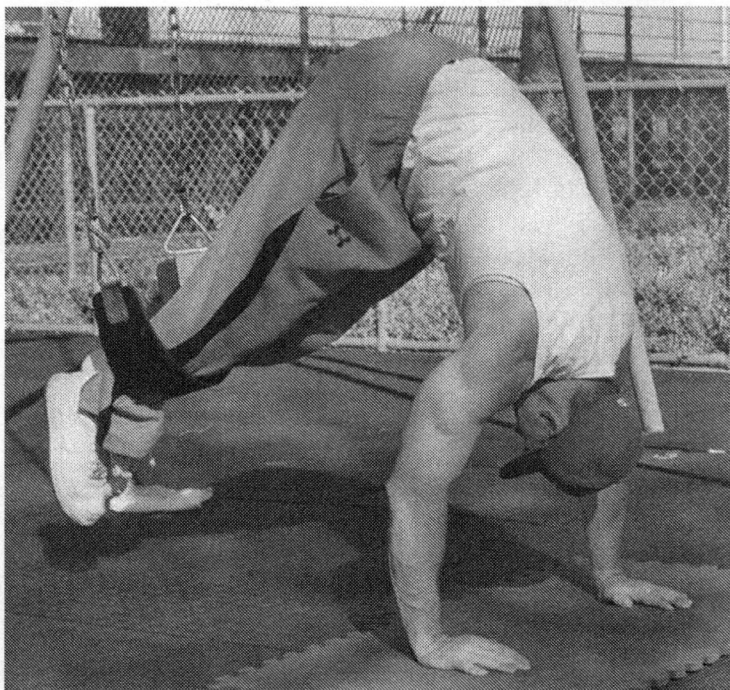

Always keep safety in mind!

Chest and Shoulders

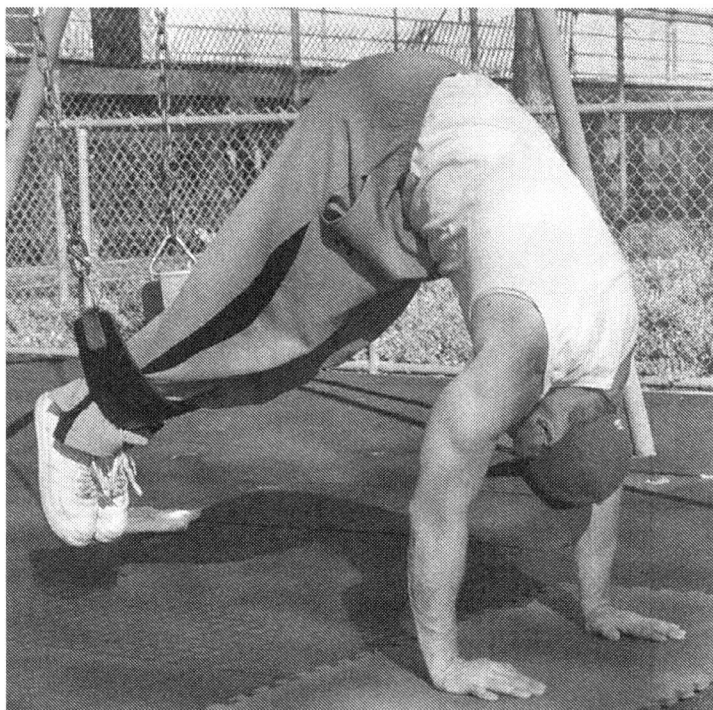

Swing Set Workouts

Push Up Alternate Lifts - Shins on Swing

Start with your back facing the swing. Place your hands on the ground. Next, place your shins / ankles on the swing. You should be in a push up / plank position with your shins on the swing. Lift your right hand and your left leg up simultaneously. Return your right hand to the ground and left leg to the swing then repeat the motion with your left hand and right leg. Your arms and legs remain straight. Keep your back straight and core muscles tight. Repeat the alternate lifts for the desired number of repetitions. You should feel this in your core muscles.

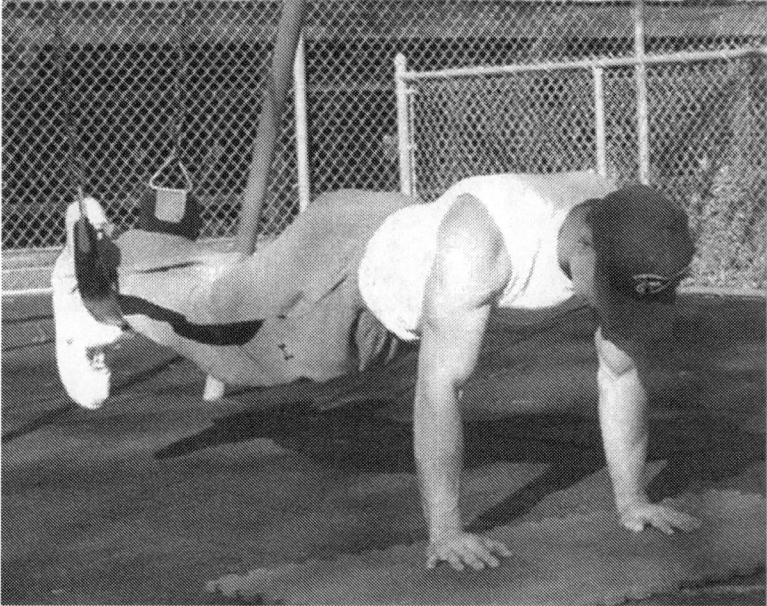

Always keep safety in mind!

Chest and Shoulders

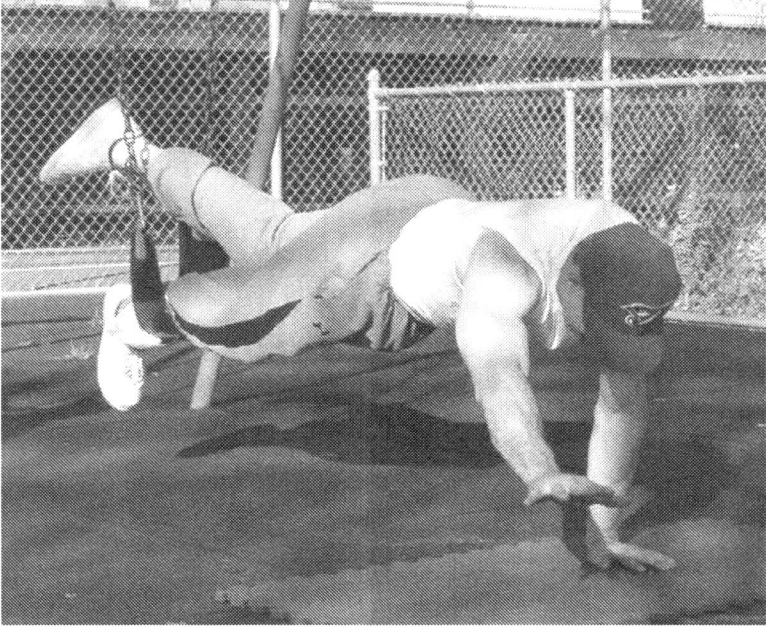

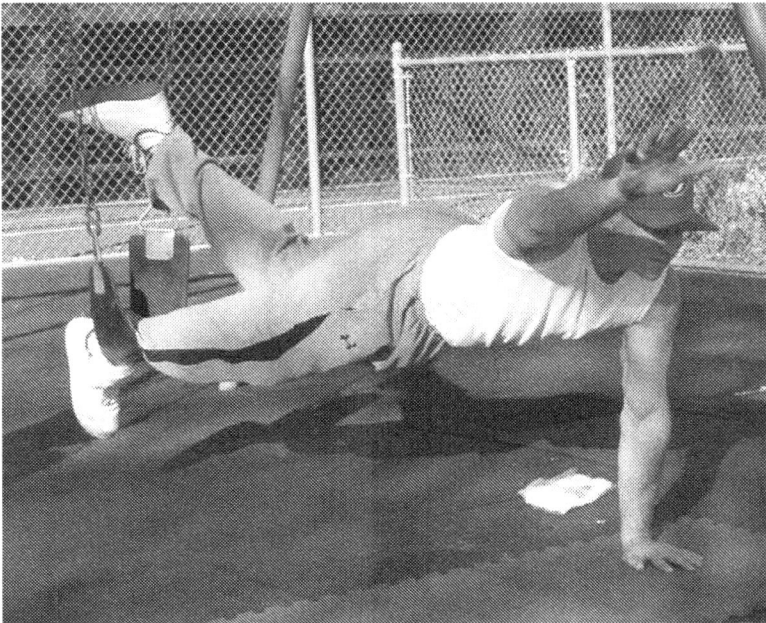

Legs and Core

This is an advanced workout. It is for people who train each body area one time per week using split routines.

Three sets per exercise are recommended and 10-15 repetitions per set are appropriate for this type of workout. Perform no more than four sets per exercise.

Swing Set Workouts

Always keep safety in mind!

Legs and Core

Supported Leg Press

Start lying with your upper back on swing and hands on chains. Begin with your legs straight and your body at approximately a 45 degree angle. Your body should be in a straight line form head to toe. Once positioned, bend your knees until they form a 90 degree angle. Your upper body continues to be supported by the swing. Make sure your knees remain in line with your hips. Do not allow your knees to fall toward each other. Make sure your knees do not go forward beyond your toes. Straighten and bend your knees for the desired number of repetitions.

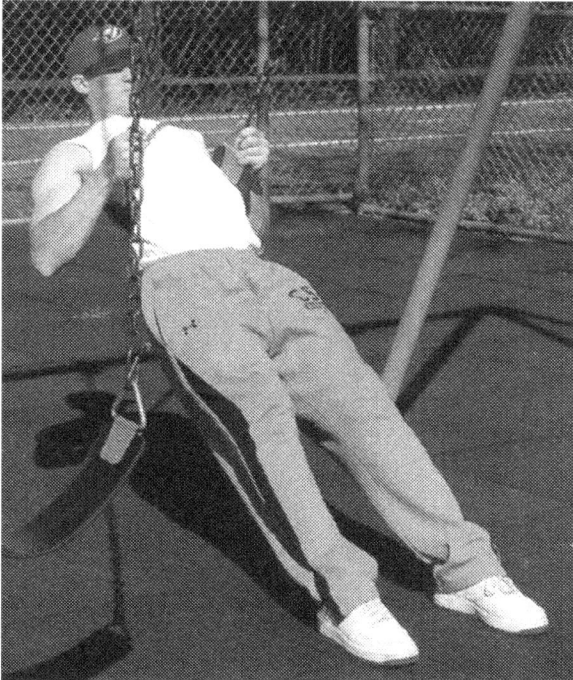

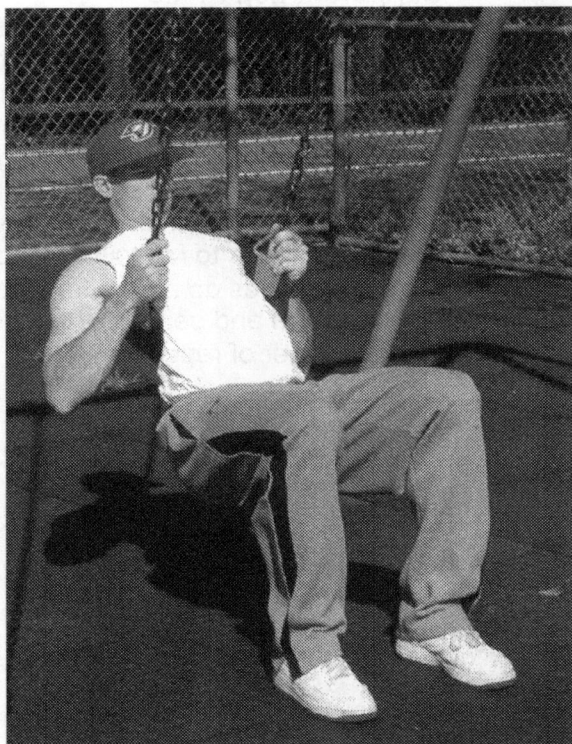

Always keep safety in mind!

Legs and Core

Single Leg Supported Leg Press

Start lying with your upper back on swing and hands on chains. Begin with your legs straight and your body at approximately a 45 degree angle. Your body should be in a straight line form head to toe. Once positioned, lift your right leg and cross it over your left leg at the knee. Once your legs are crossed, bend your left leg to form a 90 degree angle and then straighten it. Your upper body continues to be supported by the swing. Make sure your knee remains in line with your hips. Do not allow your knees to wobble side to side. Make sure your knees do not go forward beyond your toes. Straighten and bend your knee for the desired number of repetitions. Repeat this exercise for the same number of repetitions with the other leg.

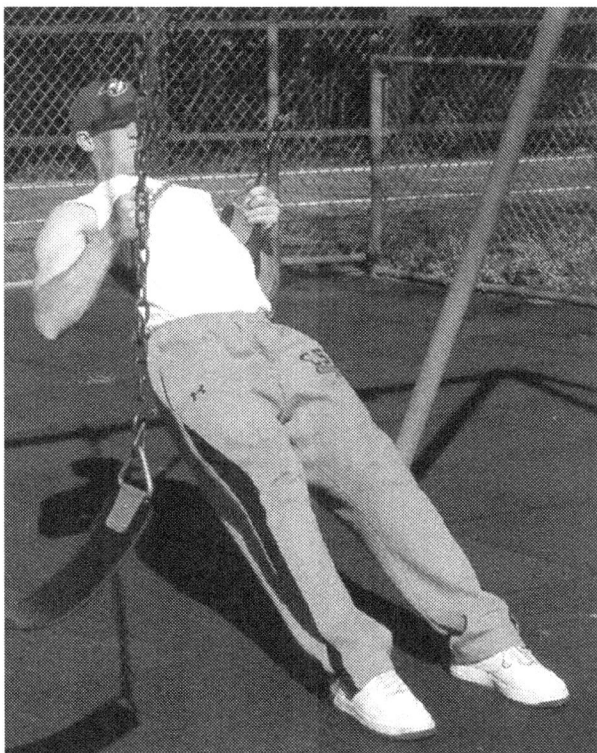

Swing Set Workouts

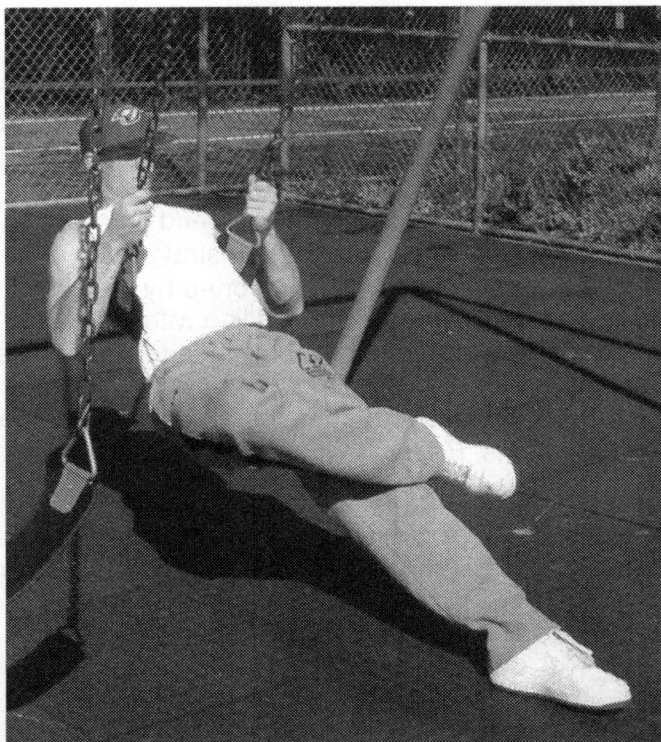

Always keep safety in mind!

Legs and Core

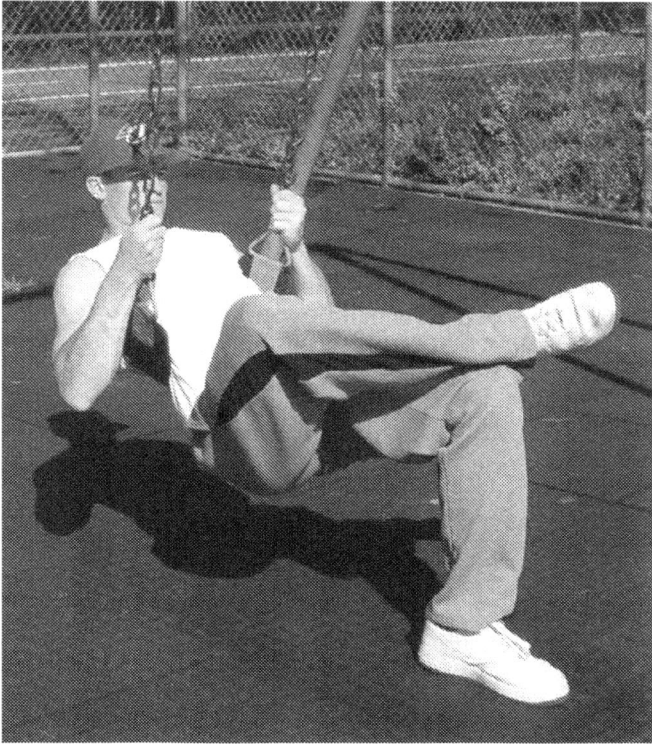

Bulgarian Squat

Start with your back facing the swing. Lift your right foot up behind your body to place your right shin on the swing. Allow the swing to slightly move backward. Once you are balanced with your right shin on the swing, bend your left leg to perform a single leg squat. Make sure you keep your left knee in line with the hip and the toes on that side. Make sure you do not allow your knee to move forward, beyond your toes. Keep your chest up throughout the exercise.

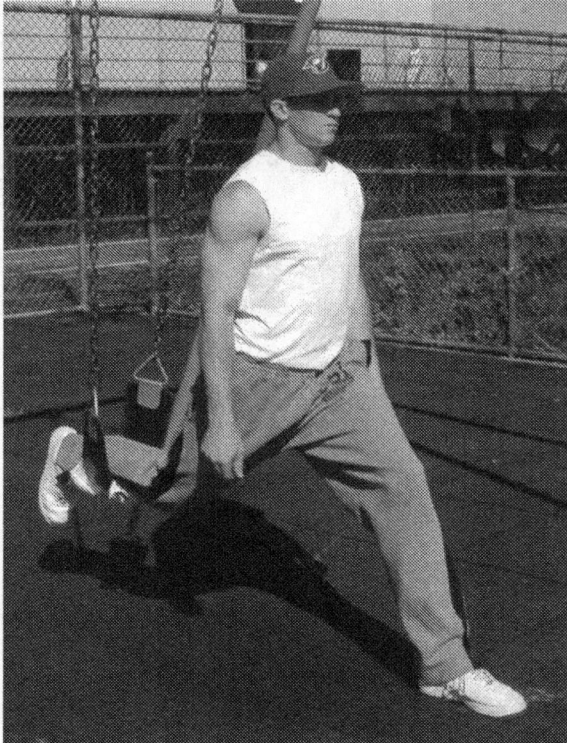

Always keep safety in mind!

Legs and Core

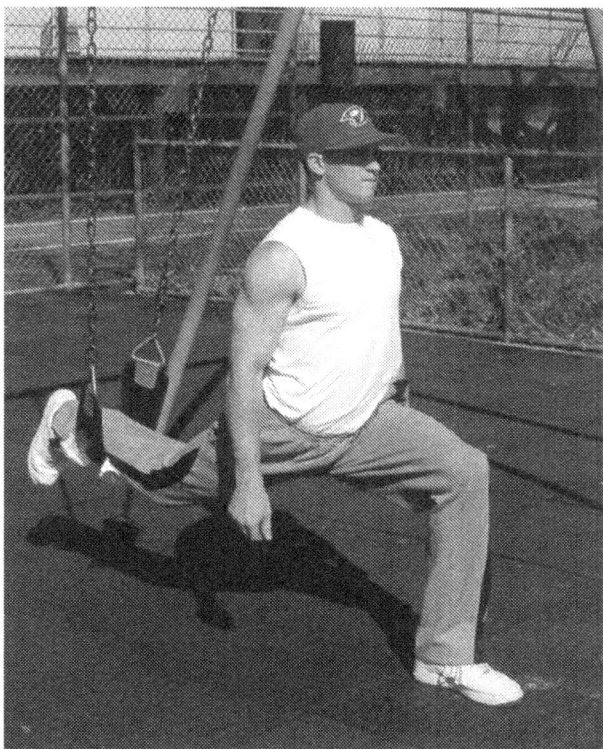

Swing Set Workouts

Knee In Tuck – Arms on Swing

Grasp the swing with both hands and position forearms on the swing. Keep your fingers wrapped around the bottom of the swing. Walk your feet backwards so that you are in a push / plank position with your forearms on the swing. Start with your body straight. Next, lift your right foot off the ground and bring your knee toward your chest, bending at the hips to form a tuck position with that leg. Return to the straight push / plank position. Repeat the single knee tuck for the desired number of repetitions. Perform this exercise with the left leg. You should feel this in your core and hip flexor muscles.

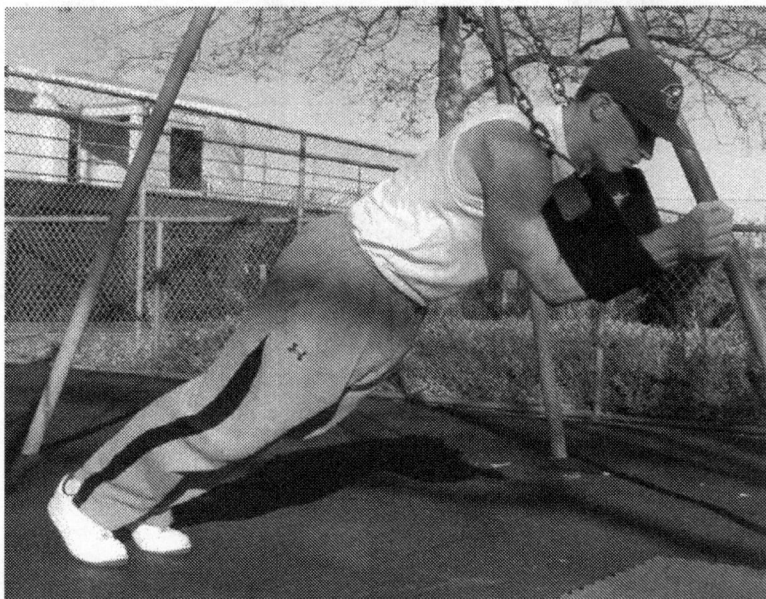

Always keep safety in mind!

Legs and Core

Foot does not touch ground in front.

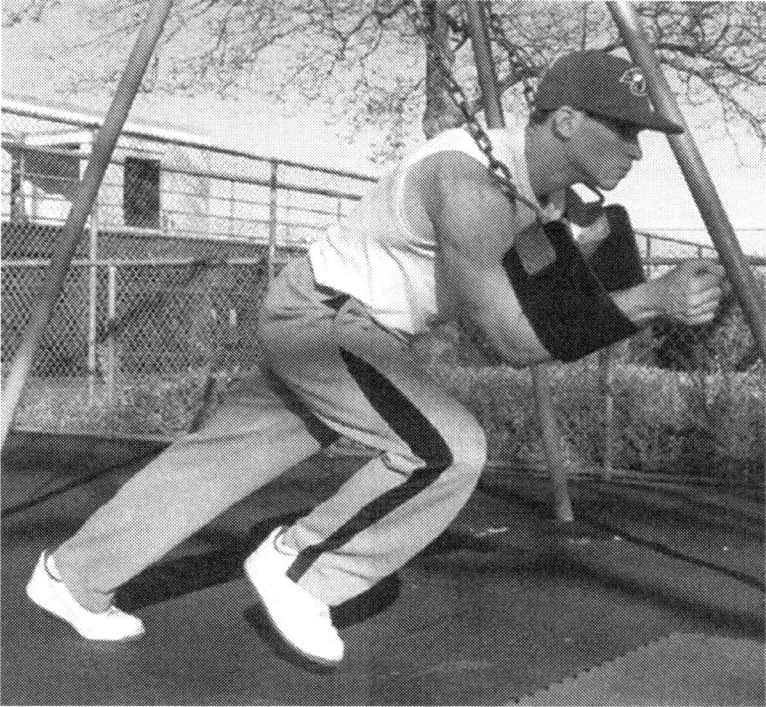

Swing Set Workouts

Swing Runners

Grasp the swing with both hands and position forearms on the swing. Keep your fingers wrapped around the bottom of the swing. Walk your feet backwards so that you are in a push / plank position with your forearms on the swing. Start with your body straight. Next, lift your right foot off the ground and bring your knee toward your chest, bending at the hips to form a tuck position with that leg. As you return right foot to the ground, quickly bring the left knee in. Continue to switch feet as if you are running with your forearms on the swing. Repeat the climbing / running motion for the desired number of repetitions. You should feel this in your core, hip flexor, and quadriceps muscles. Make sure you do not slam your heel toward the ground because it would force your foot to flex too much. Remain on the balls of your foot while running.

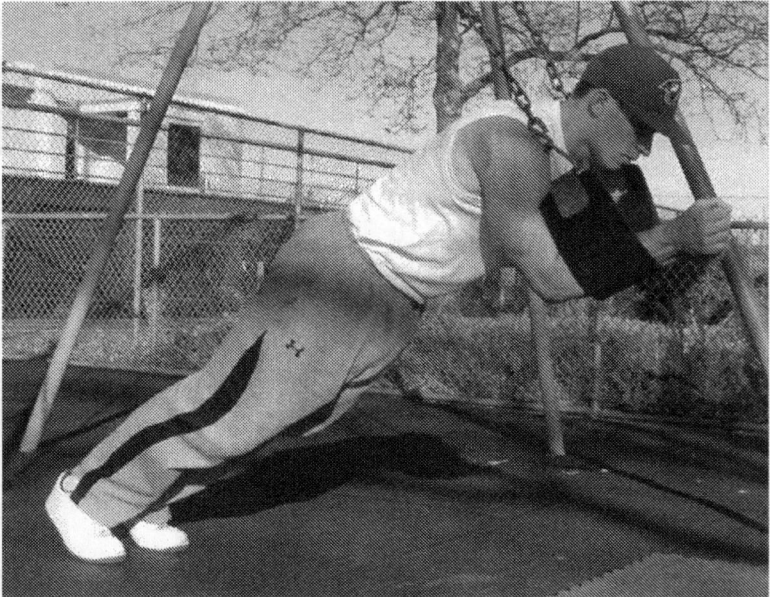

Always keep safety in mind!

Legs and Core

Foot does not touch ground in front.

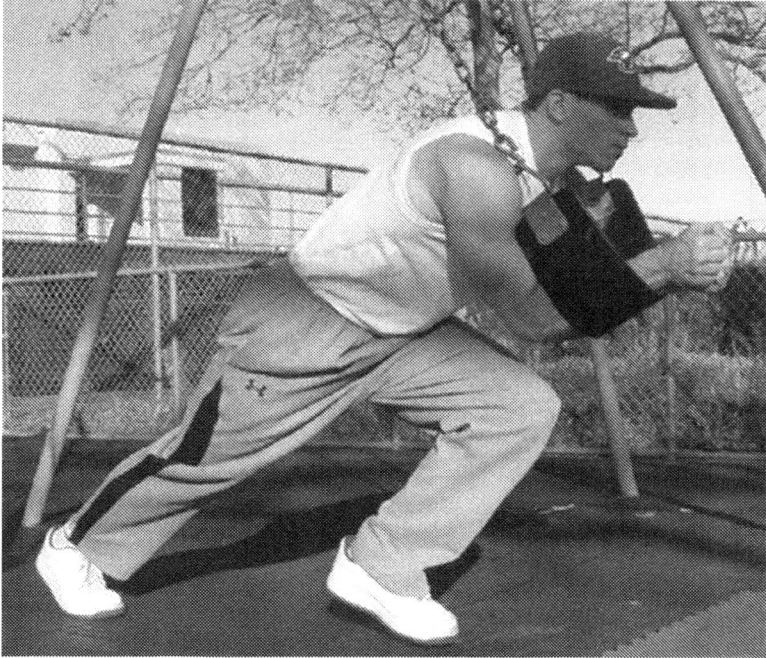

Swing Set Workouts

Foot does not touch ground in front.

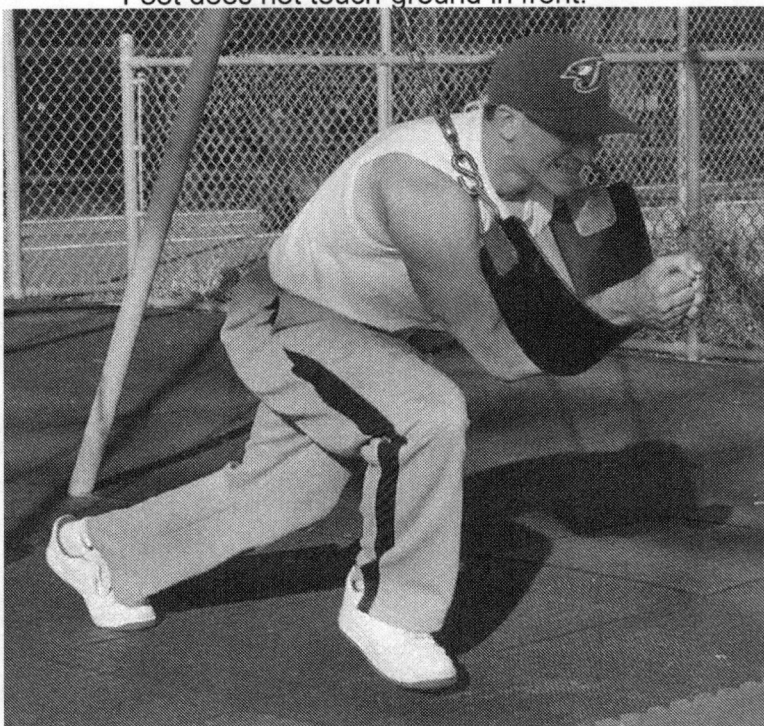

Always keep safety in mind!

Oblique – Straight Body

Sit on the swing, hold the chains, and lean back. Lift both legs to hip / swing height. Next, roll over toward your right hip so that your belly faces the left chain. Once both legs are straight and you are facing the chain, use your core / oblique muscles to slightly lift your legs toward the sky. Simultaneously lift your shoulders toward the sky. The lifts should be small and continuous. Return your legs to the starting position and then perform the lift again. Perform this exercise with your belly facing the left. Continue to perform side lifts for the desired number of repetitions. Keep your legs nearly straight throughout the exercise. You should feel this in your side, your oblique muscles.

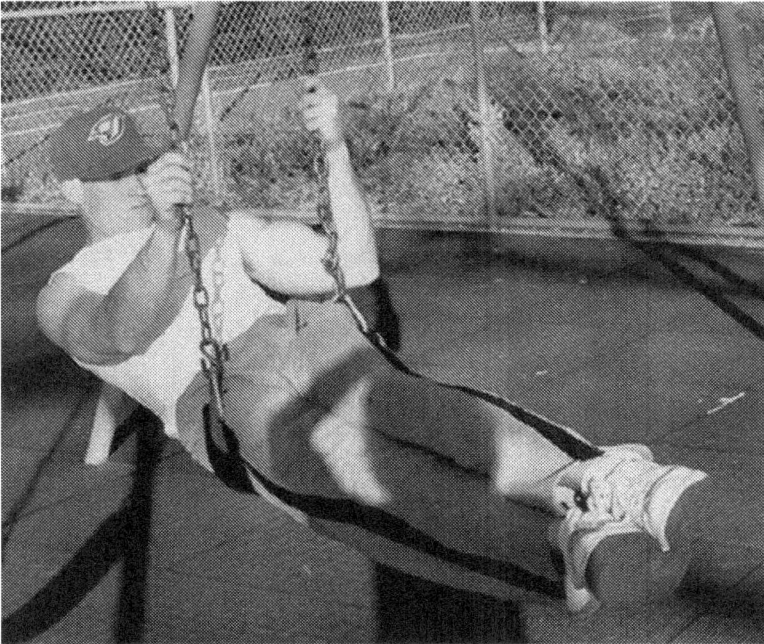

Swing Set Workouts

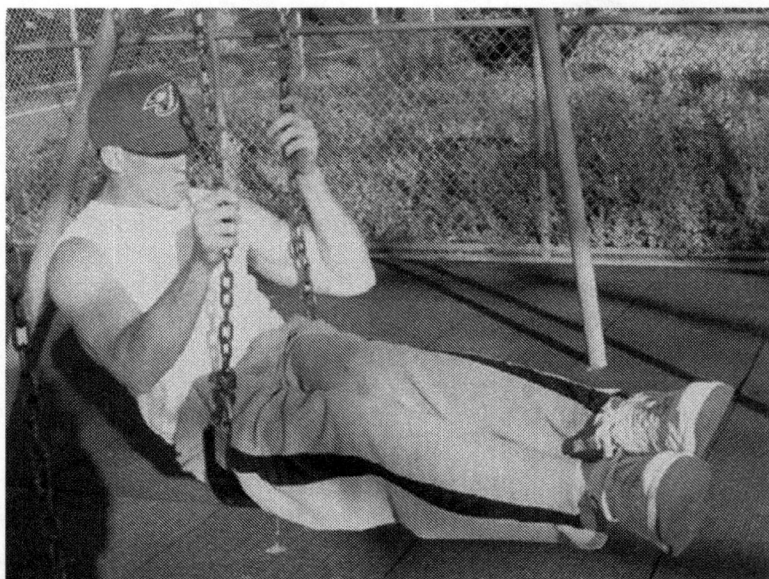

Always keep safety in mind!

Legs and Core

Oblique Crunch – Knees Bent

Sit on the swing, hold the chains, and lean back. Lift both legs to hip / swing height. Next, roll over toward your right hip so that your belly faces the left chain. Once both legs are bent and at hip height, lift them up and toward your left armpit. Return your legs to the starting position. Continue to perform side bent knee crunches for the desired number of repetitions. You should feel this in your side, your oblique muscles.

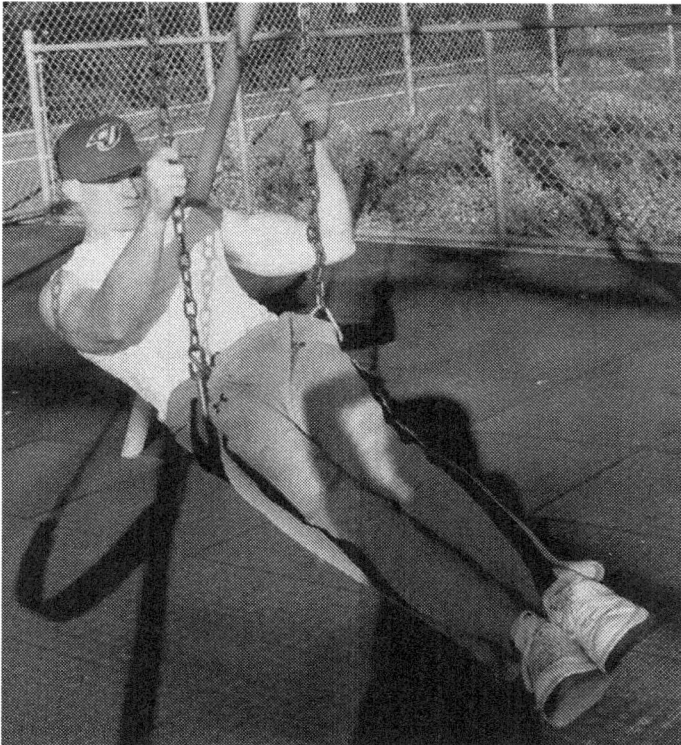

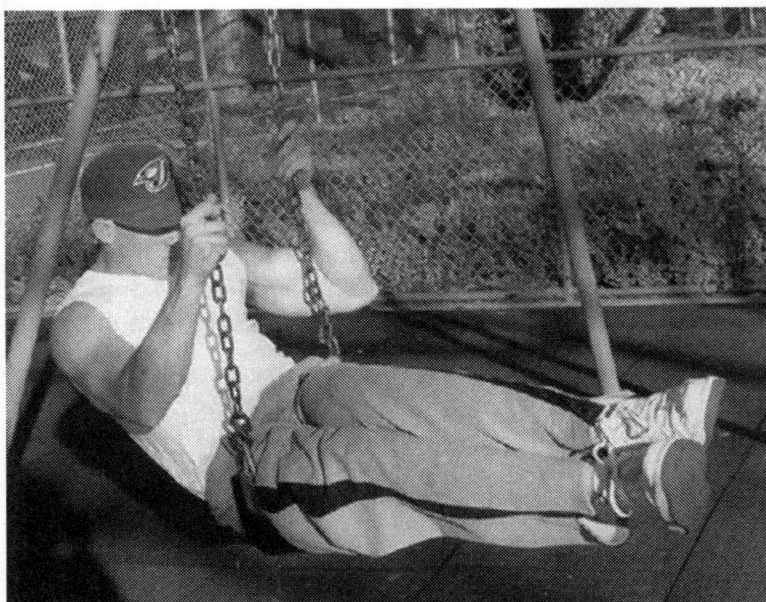

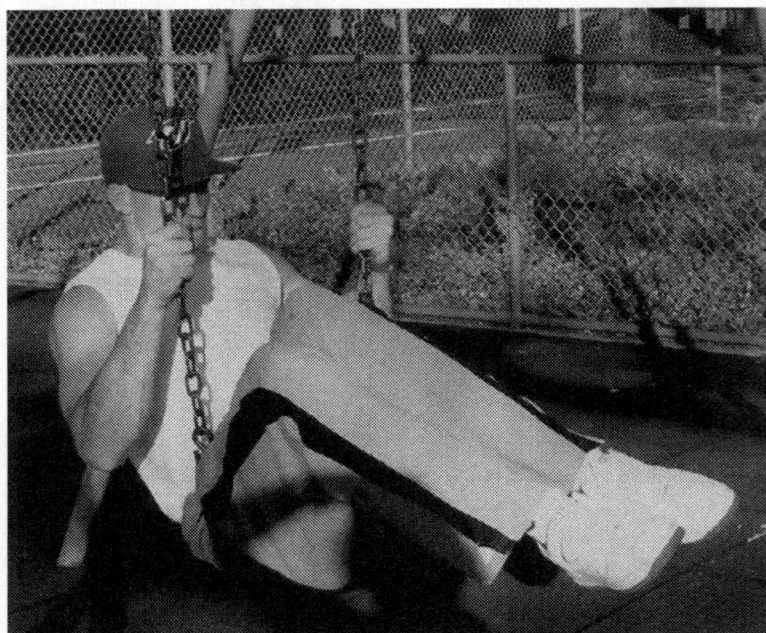

Always keep safety in mind!

Legs and Core

Double Crunch

Sit on the swing, hold the chains, and lean back. Lift both legs in front of your body to hip /swing height. Once both legs are at hip / swing height, bring both knees in toward your chest together. As you bring your knees in toward your chest, sit up to allow your chest and knees to meet. Once your knees and chest have formed a tuck position, return to the starting position. Continue to bring your knees in and chest up for the desired number of repetitions. You should feel this in your abdominal and hip flexor muscles.

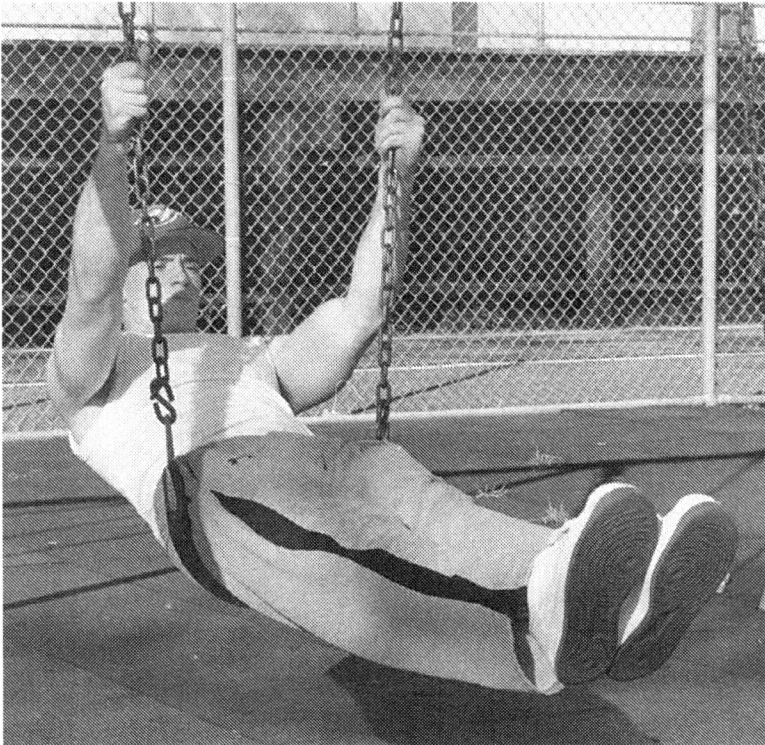

Swing Set Workouts

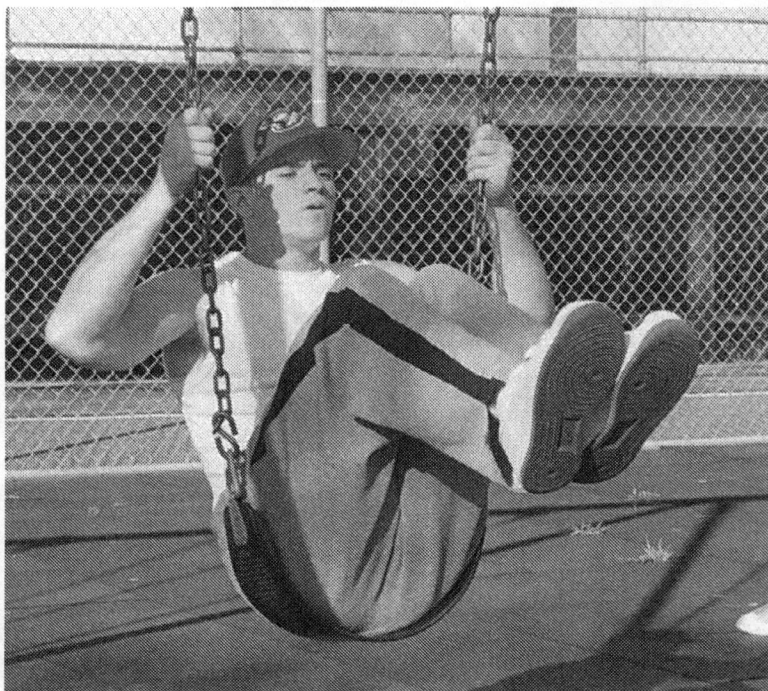

Always keep safety in mind!

V-Up on Swing
Sit on the swing, hold the chains, and lean back. Keeping your legs straight, lift them in front of your body to hip / swing height. Once both legs are at hip / swing height, simultaneously lift both legs up toward your chest. As you bring your thighs in toward your chest, sit up to allow your chest and thighs to meet. Once your knees and chest have formed a V or tight pike position, return to the extended seated position. Continue to bring your legs and chest up for the desired number of repetitions. You should feel this in your abdominal and hip flexor muscles.

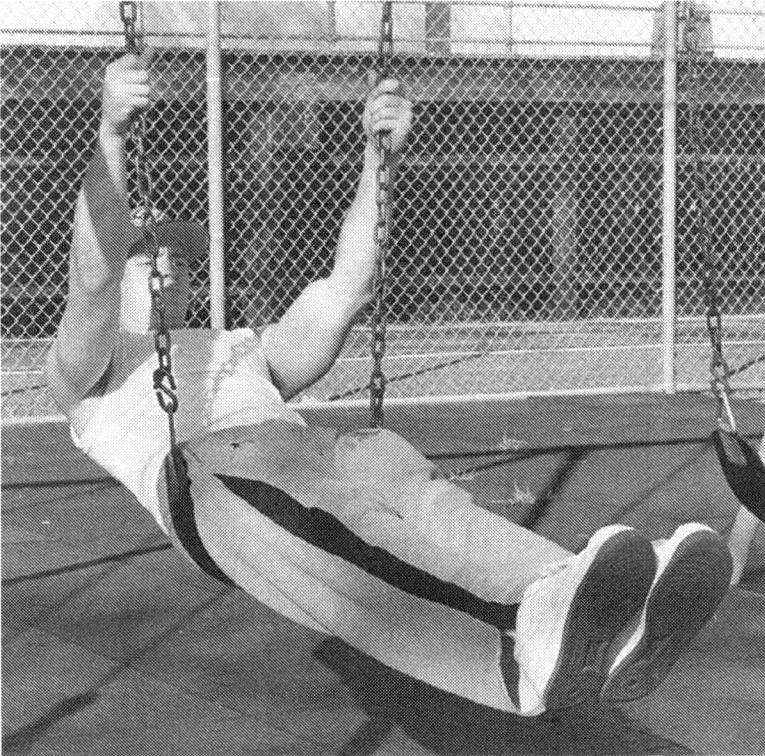

Swing Set Workouts

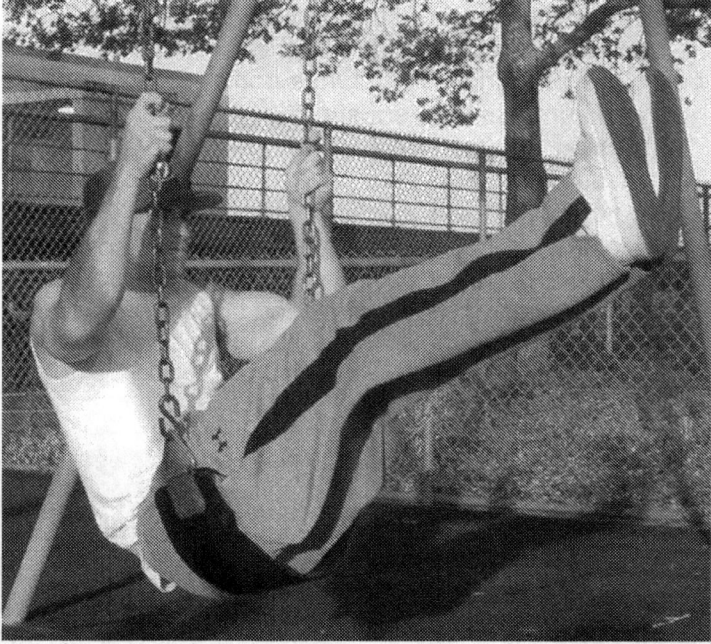

Always keep safety in mind!

Legs and Core

Alternating Single Leg V-Up
Sit on the swing, hold the chains, and lean back. Keeping your legs straight, lift them in front of your body to hip / swing height. Once both legs are at hip / swing height, lift your right leg up toward your chest. As you bring your right thigh in toward your chest, sit up to allow your chest and thigh to meet. Once your right leg and chest have formed a V or tight pike position, return the right leg to the extended position, lean back, then perform the single leg V-Up with the left leg. Continue to alternate the single leg lift to the V position for the desired number of repetitions. Keep your legs straight throughout the exercise. You should feel this in your abdominal and hip flexor muscles

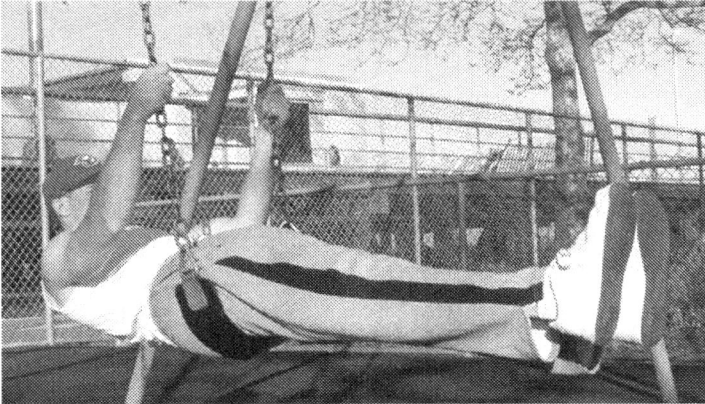

Swing Set Workouts

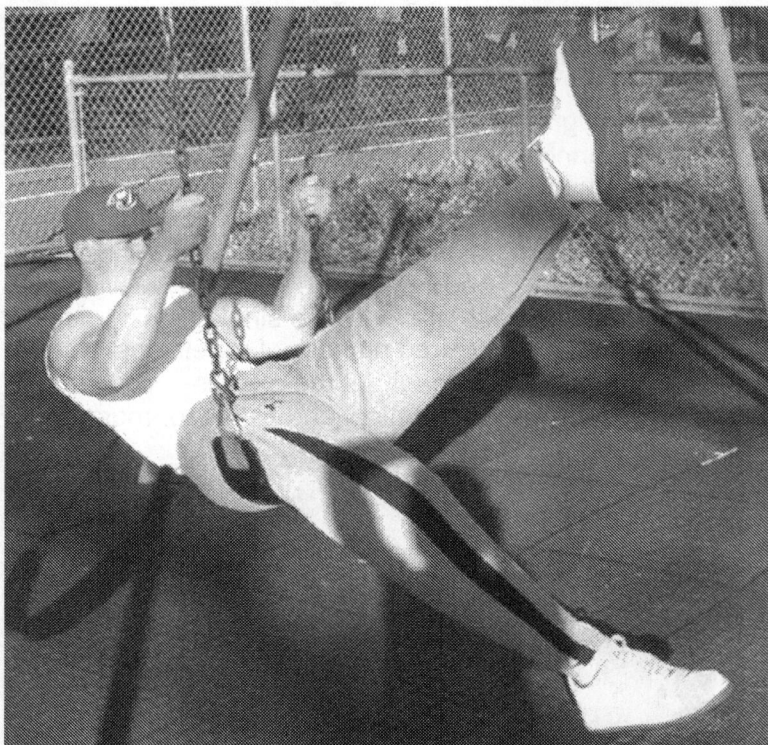

Always keep safety in mind!

Legs and Core 2

This is an advanced workout. It is for people who train each body area one time per week using split routines.

Three sets per exercise are recommended and 10-15 repetitions per set are appropriate for this type of workout. Perform no more than four sets per exercise.

Swing Set Workouts

Always keep safety in mind!

Squat – Hold Swing (Lean Back)

Start facing the swing. Grasp the outer portion of the swing with both hands and wrap fingers over the swing. (Other option is to grasp the lowest portion of the chains.) Holding the swing securely, lean backward and walk your feet forward so that you are at approximately a 45 degree angle. Make sure your feet will not slide. Keep your chest up and bend both knees to perform a squat. Make sure your knees remain in line with your hips. Do not allow your knees to fall toward each other. Make sure your knees do not go forward beyond your toes. Straighten and bend your knees for the desired number of repetitions.

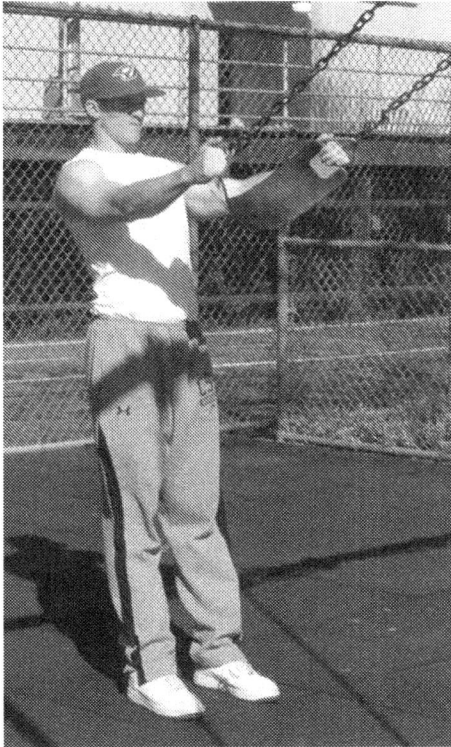

Swing Set Workouts

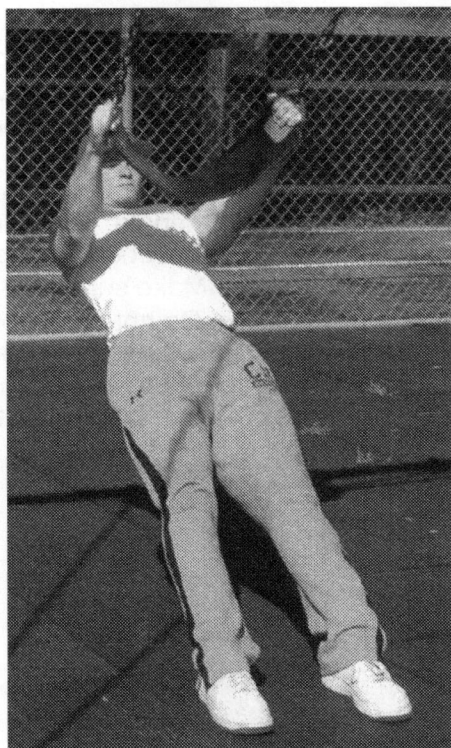

Always keep safety in mind!

Legs and Core 2

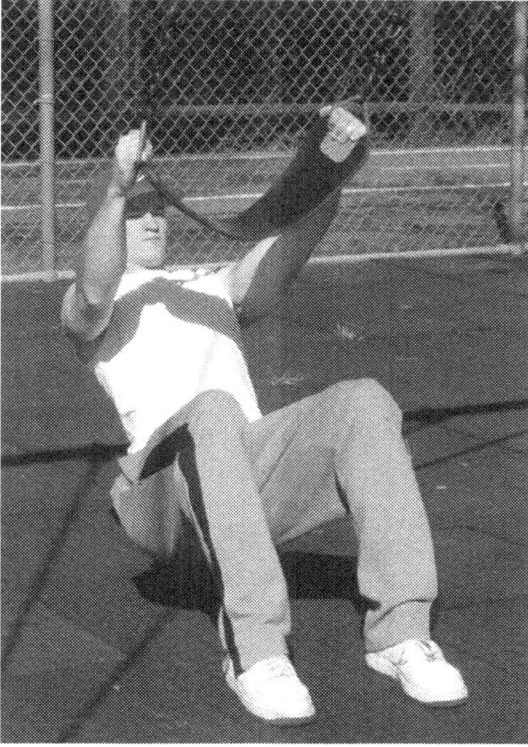

Step Up

Start standing facing the swing. Reach up and grasp the chains, one with each hand. Lift your left leg up and place your left foot securely on the swing as if about to step up. Hold the chains securely and keep your left foot in place on the center of the swing. Step up onto the swing. Bring the toes of your right foot to the edge of the swing and immediately return the right foot to the ground. The swing will move forward and back as you step up and down. This will be a very quick rhythmic motion. Step up and down before the seat of the swing returns to the start position. Be very careful with foot placement when returning the supporting foot to the ground.

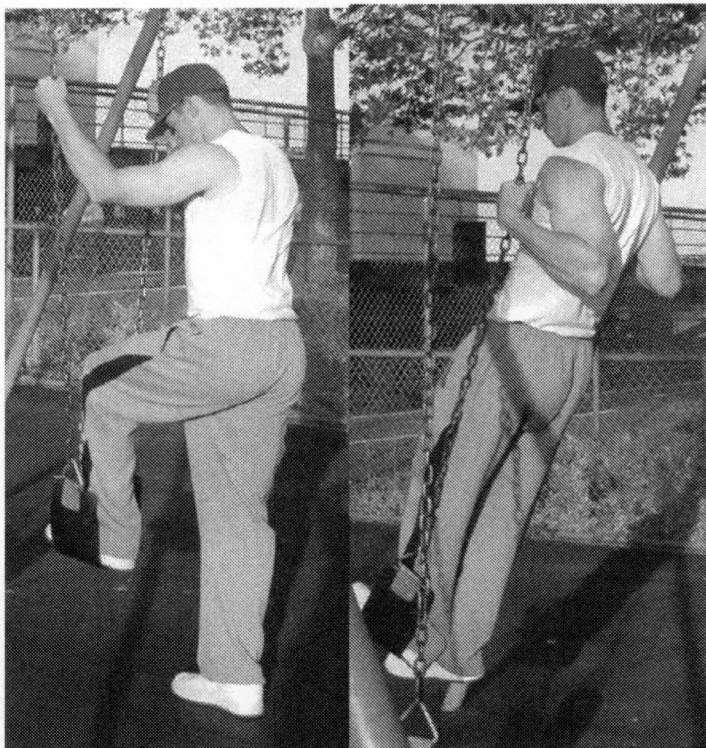

Always keep safety in mind!

Legs and Core 2

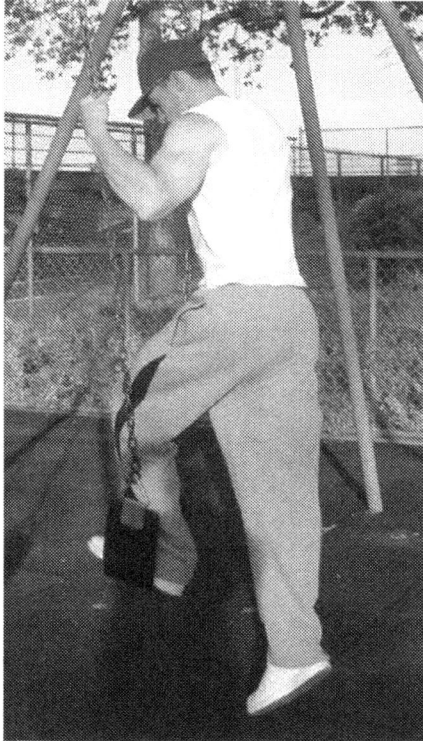

Bulgarian Squat
Start with your back facing the swing. Lift your right foot up behind your body to place your right shin on the swing. Once you are balanced with your right shin on the swing, bend your left leg to perform a single leg squat. Make sure you keep your left knee in line with the hip and the toes on that side. Make sure you do not allow your knee to move forward, beyond your toes. Keep your chest up throughout the exercise.

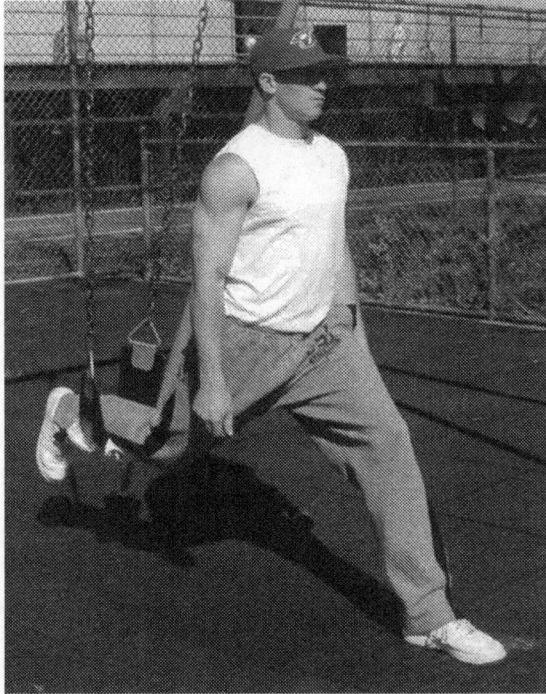

Legs and Core 2

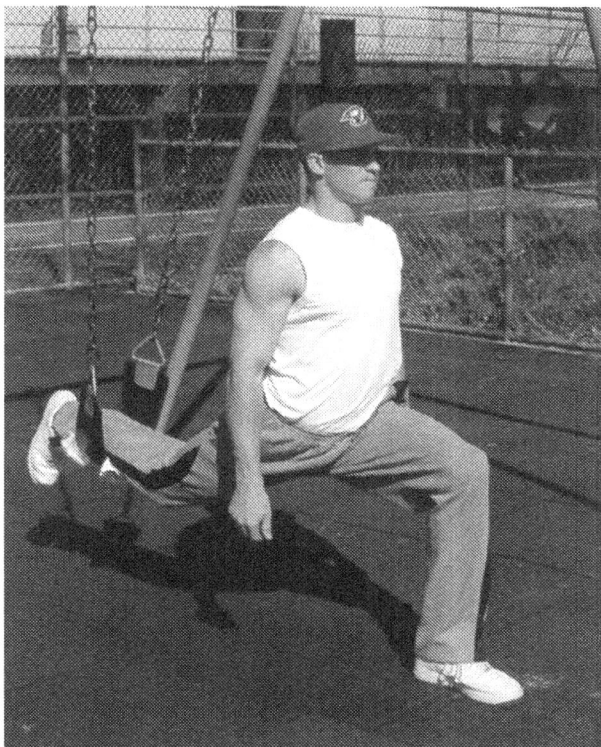

Swing Set Workouts

Lunge - Step Back

Start facing the swing. Grasp the outer portion of the swing with both hands and wrap fingers over the swing. Keeping your fingers wrapped around the bottom of the swing, step backward with your right leg and lower that knee toward the ground. Do not allow the knee or foot to touch the ground. Think of leaning back as you lunge. Lift off the ground using the quadriceps in the left leg and return to the starting position. Keep your chest up throughout the exercise. Make sure you keep your supporting knee in line with your hip and the toes on that side. Make sure you do not allow your knee to bend greater than a 90 degree angle.

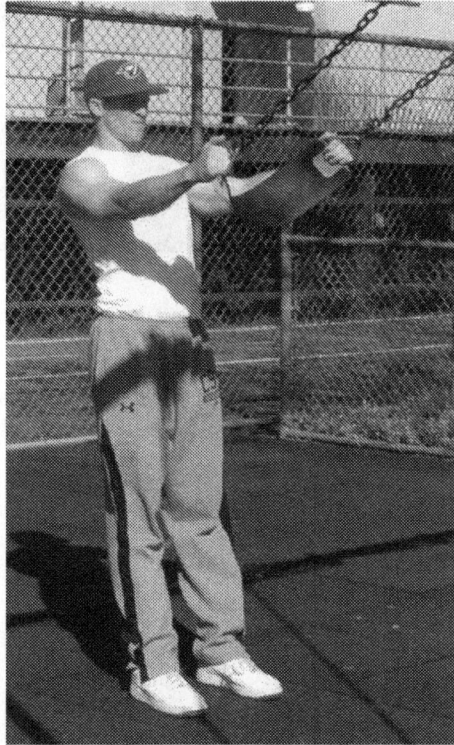

Always keep safety in mind!

Legs and Core 2

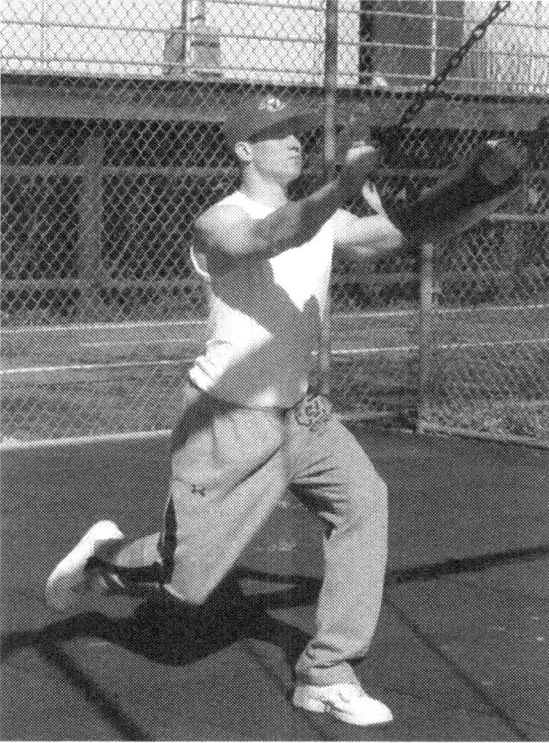

Swing Set Workouts

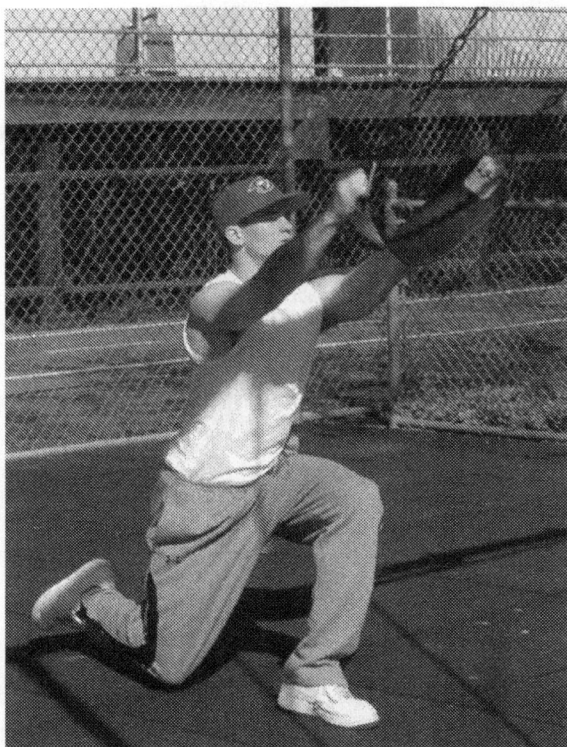

Always keep safety in mind!

Legs and Core 2

Knee In Tuck – Arms on Swing

Grasp the swing with both hands and position forearms on the swing. Keep your fingers wrapped around the bottom of the swing. Walk your feet backwards so that you are in a push / plank position with your forearms on the swing. Start with your body straight. Next, lift your right foot off the ground and bring your knee toward your chest, bending at the hips to form a tuck position with that leg. Return to the straight push / plank position. Repeat the single knee tuck for the desired number of repetitions. Perform this exercise with the left leg. You should feel this in your core and hip flexor muscles.

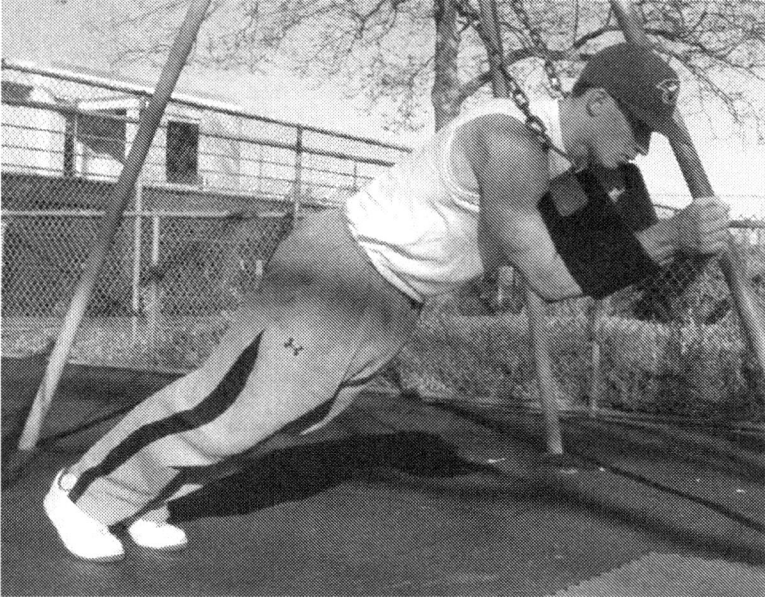

Swing Set Workouts

Foot does not touch ground in front.

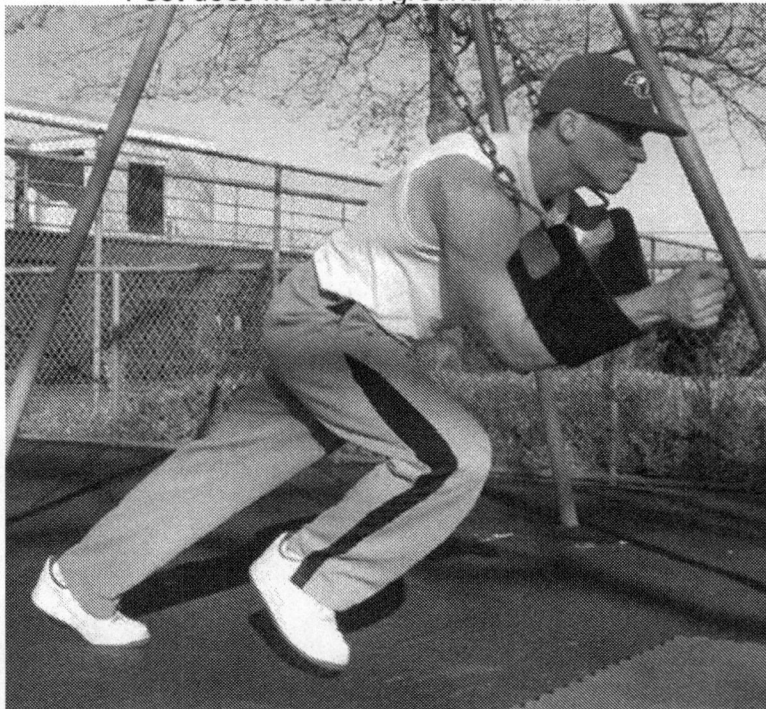

Always keep safety in mind!

Legs and Core 2

Alternate the Flutter Kicks with the V-Ups. Perform 10 Flutter Kicks, 10 V-Ups, 10 Flutter Kicks, and 10 V-Ups. This will give you 40 repetitions, nonstop.

Flutter Kicks

Sit on the swing, hold the chains, and lean back. Keeping your legs straight, lift them in front of your body to hip / swing height. Once both legs are at hip / swing height, lift your right leg up 6-8 inches. Next, simultaneously return the right leg to hip / swing height and lift the left leg 6-8 inches off the swing. Continue to perform very quick alternating low lifts for the desired number of repetitions. Keep your legs straight throughout the exercise. You should feel this in your abdominal and hip flexor muscles.

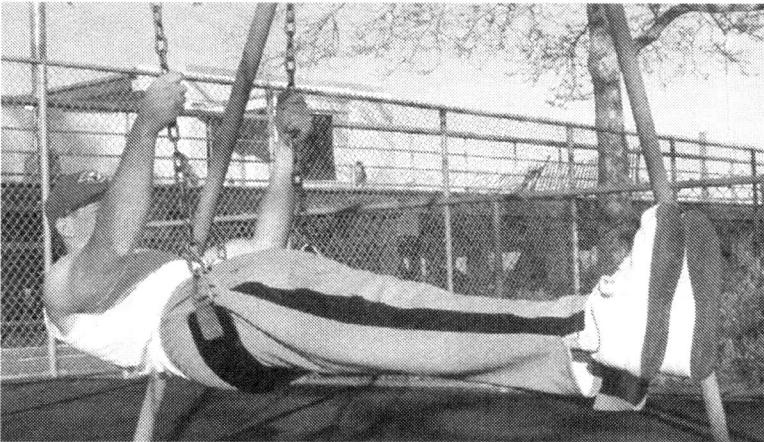

Swing Set Workouts

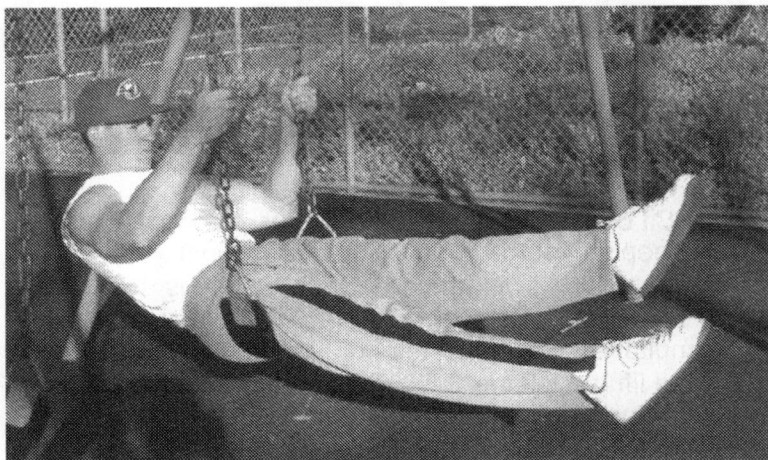

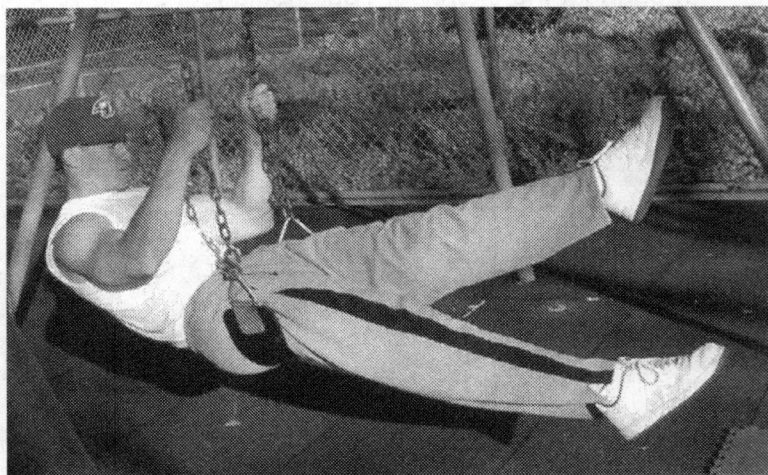

Always keep safety in mind!

Legs and Core 2

V-Up on Swing

Sit on the swing, hold the chains, and lean back. Keeping your legs straight, lift them in front of your body to hip / swing height. Once both legs are at hip / swing height, simultaneously lift both legs up toward your chest. As you bring your thighs in toward your chest, sit up to allow your chest and thighs to meet. Once your knees and chest have formed a V or tight pike position, return to the extended seated position. Continue to bring your legs and chest up for the desired number of repetitions. You should feel this in your abdominal and hip flexor muscles.

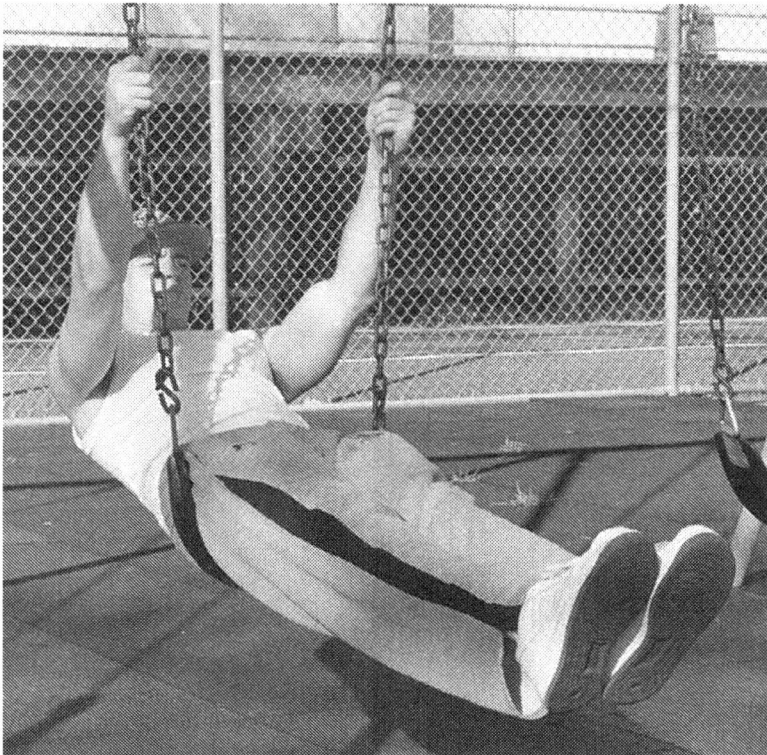

Swing Set Workouts

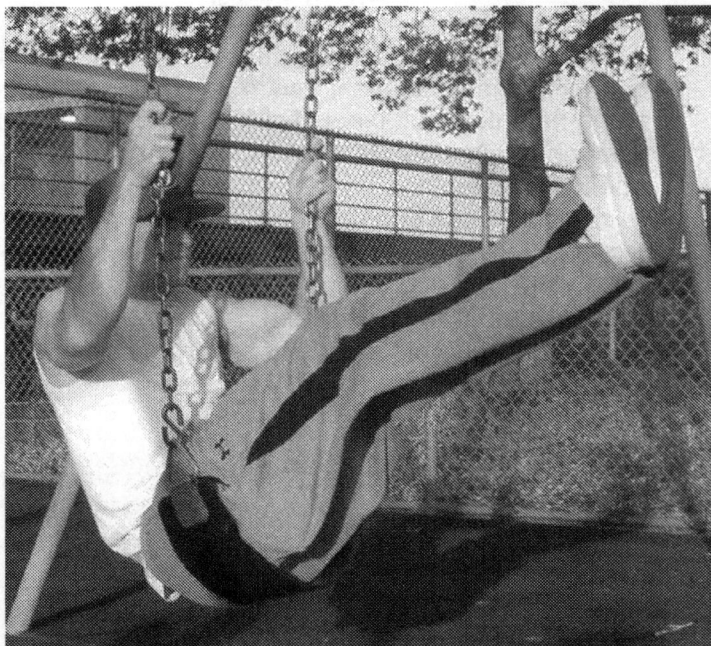

Always keep safety in mind!

Quad Stretch Stand Hold Foot

Start out standing next to the swing set base. Grasp the base with your left hand. Bend your right leg and bring your right foot toward your buttocks. With your right hand grasp your ankle and then pull your right heel in toward your buttocks until you feel a gentle stretch in your right quadriceps muscles. Hold the stretch for approximately 20 seconds. Repeat this exercise stretching your left leg.

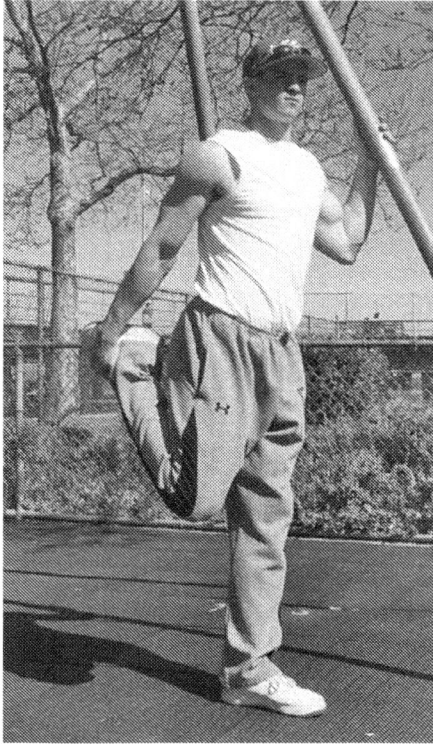

Hamstring Stretch (1 Foot on Swing)

Start standing facing the seat of the swing. Lift your right leg up and place your right heel on the swing. Once your heel is on the swing, grasp the chains for balance. Keep your heel on the swing and bend at your hip, leaning in toward your leg. Keep your back straight so that you feel the stretch in your hamstring muscles. Many people will feel this stretch without leaning forward. For a more intense stretch, flex your foot so that your toes point up toward the sky. Do not lock your knee in this stretch. Hold this stretch for approximately 20 seconds. Repeat this exercise with your left leg.

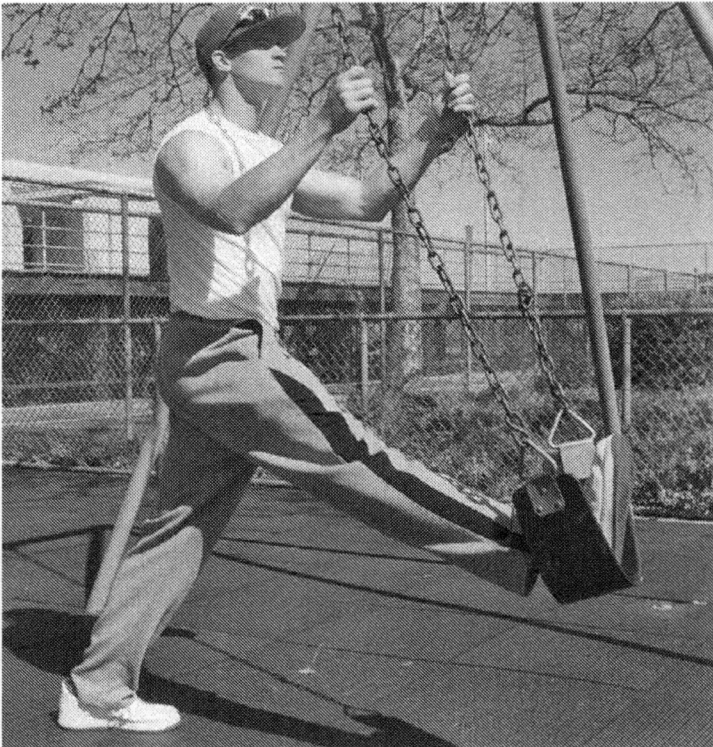

Legs and Core 2

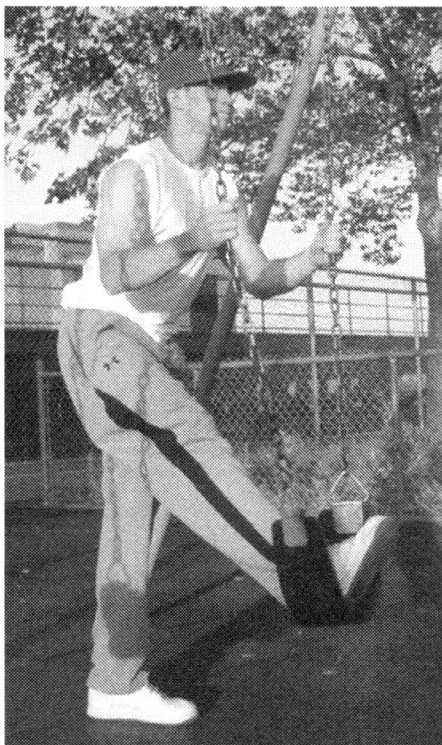

About Karen Goeller

Karen Goeller's gymnastics career spans over 30 years, as a gymnast, gymnastics coach, gymnastics facility owner, and as a published author.

This amazing author has written more gymnastics books than any one person in the USA with sales worldwide. She has helped educate thousands in the gymnastics community as a coach and writer. Her books are currently used by gymnastics coaches, fitness experts, and physical education teachers among many other professionals.

Karen Goeller's published works include the famous gymnastics drills and conditioning books, gymnastics and fitness journals, a gymnastics parent's guide, and several fitness training programs.

Karen Goeller has had gymnastics articles published in USA Gymnastics Technique Magazine and on various websites. Her articles include, "The Handstand is the Most Important Skill," "Ahh...The Glide Kip," "Fun with Running, a Crucial Skill", and "Cast Handstand" among others.

Before her success as a published author, Karen Goeller owned and operated a gymnastics club in NYC for 10 years, worked for the most famous gymnastics coach, Bela Karolyi, worked at International Gymnastics Camp for a decade of holiday clinics, and worked at various health clubs in NYC.

Before she earned her BA Degree, Karen Goeller's studies included Physical Therapy, Health Sciences, Nutrition, and Emergency Medical Care. She has held certifications such as a NY State EMT, Nutritional

Swing Set Workouts

Analysis, Fitness Trainer, Counseling Techniques, Childcare Fundamentals, USA Gymnastics Safety, USA Gymnastics Skill Evaluator, and USA Gymnastics Meet Director, among many others.

Besides being author to this book, Karen Goeller was one of two photographers.

Special thanks to Steven Porter, contributing photographer. He has captured scenic views, special moments, and action shots. Much of his work has been featured on posters, t-shirts, mugs, and other gift items sold through PortersGifts.com.

Other Books by Karen Goeller

Fitness on a Swing Set
ISBN: 9780615147888

Gymnastics Drills and Conditioning Exercises
ISBN: 9781411605794

Gymnastics Drills and Conditioning for the Handstand
ISBN: 9781411650008

Gymnastics Drills: Walkover, Limber, and Back Handspring
ISBN: 9781411611603

Gymnastics Conditioning for the Legs and Ankles
ISBN: 9781411620339

Gymnastics Journal: My Scores, My Goals, My Dreams
ISBN: 9781411641457

The Most Frequently Asked Questions about Gymnastics
ISBN: 1591133726

Fitness Journal: Goals, Training, and Success
ISBN: 9781847284440

Strength Training Journal
ISBN: 9780615147598

Gymnastics Conditioning: Five Conditioning Workouts
ISBN: Not yet assigned.

Gymnastics Conditioning: Tumbling Conditioning
ISBN: Not yet assigned.

www.GymnasticsBooks.com

About Brian Dowd

For Brian Dowd, this is his first contribution to a published work. He was the one who carefully tested more than 50 exercises to make sure they really could be transferred to a swing. That same day Brian Dowd also worked as the fitness model for this project. He posed several times for each exercise to help ensure the photo was not only captured, but that his form was technically correct.

Brian Dowd's sport has always been baseball. He has been a member of numerous travel baseball teams growing up and competed in the AAU, NABF, AABC National Championships, and the AAU Junior Olympics National Championships among others. Brian also played 4 years of varsity baseball for one of the best and most respected high school programs in New York City. After high school, Brian went on to play 4 years of NCAA College Baseball and now plays semi-professional baseball in the New York area. Brian Dowd currently coaches the high school team he once played for in New York City.

This amazing baseball player has learned a great deal about fitness and sports conditioning throughout the years and has now made a major contribution to the completion of these highly useful fitness books.

Swing Set Workouts

Always keep safety in mind!

www.ingramcontent.com/pod-product-compliance
Lightning Source LLC
Chambersburg PA
CBHW031505270326
41930CB00006B/257